LOOK GREAT NAKED

SLIM DOWN,
SHAPE UP AND TONE YOUR
TROUBLE ZONES IN JUST
15 MINUTES A DAY

BRAD SCHOENFELD

Foreword by
CAROLE SEMPLE-MARZETTA 1997 Fitness Olympia Champion

Prentice
Hall Press

Library of Congress Cataloging-in-Publication Data

Schoenfeld, Brad
   Look great naked : slim down, shape up and tone your trouble zones
in just 15 minutes a day / by Brad Schoenfeld.
     p. cm.
   ISBN 0–7352–0230–3
   1. Reducing exercises.   2. Exercise for women.   I. Title.
RA781.6.S36 2001
646.7′5′082—dc21   00–058862

Acquisitions Editor: *Gene Brissie*
Production Editor: *Tom Curtin*
Interior Design/Layout: *Dee Coroneos*

Not all exercises or diets are suitable for everyone. Before you begin this program, you should have permission from your doctor to participate in vigorous
exercise and change of diet. If you feel discomfort or pain when you exercise,
do not continue. The instructions and advice presented are in no way intended
as a substitute for medical counseling. The author and publisher disclaim any
liability or loss in connection with the exercise and advice provided herein.

Printed in the United States of America

10 9 8 7 6 5 4 3 2

ISBN 0-7352-0230-3

ATTENTION: CORPORATIONS AND SCHOOLS

Prentice Hall Press books are available at quantity discounts with bulk purchase for
educational, business, or sales promotional use. For information, please write to:
Prentice Hall, Special Sales, 240 Frisch Court, Paramus, NJ 07652. Please supply: title
of book, ISBN, quantity, how the book will be used, date needed.

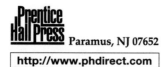 Paramus, NJ 07652

http://www.phdirect.com

ABOUT THE AUTHOR

Brad Schoenfeld, CSCS, CPT, is a renowned expert on fitness and sports nutrition. As the owner/operator of the exclusive Personal Training Center for Women in Scarsdale, New York, he is regarded as one of the leading authorities on women's fitness.

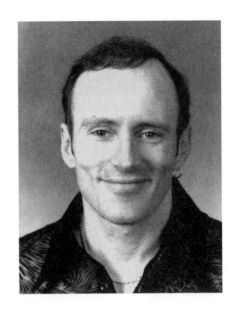

Schoenfeld is author of the best-selling fitness book, *Sculpting Her Body Perfect.* He is also a popular freelance writer on a variety of fitness topics and is a regular contributor to many leading fitness magazines including *Self, Shape, Fitness, Ms. Fitness, Oxygen,* and *Musclemag.* He has been featured on television's CBS Evening News, Good Day New York, FOX National News, and Today in New York, as well as on hundreds of radio programs across the country.

Certified as a Strength and Conditioning Specialist by the National Strength and Conditioning Association (NSCA) and as a Personal Trainer by the American Council on Exercise (ACE) and Aerobics and Fitness Association of America (AFAA), Schoenfeld is President of Global Fitness Services, a diverse, multifaceted fitness corporation. He lectures internationally on fitness, both at the corporate and consumer level.

Schoenfeld lives in Croton, New York. He may be contacted at Global Fitness Services, Box 58, Scarsdale, NY 10583.

Check out the *Look Great Naked* website at **www.lookgreatnaked.com**

ACKNOWLEDGMENTS

➡ To super-agent Bob Silverstein, for finding the proper home for this project.

➡ To Gene Brissie, for seeing the potential in this book and allocating the necessary resources to make it a success.

➡ To Dee Coroneos, for putting together the interior of the book and delivering a beautiful finished product.

➡ To the entire Prentice Hall staff, for being so friendly and helpful.

➡ To my parents, for their continual support.

➡ To all my clients at the Personal Training Center for Women, past and present, for helping me perfect the High-Energy Fitness system and furthering my quest for self-actualization.

➡ To all the trainers who have worked at the Personal Training Center for Women, past and present, for helping me make a positive impact on the lives of many.

➡ To Clarissa Chueire, Stacey Russo, Michelle Gabriele, Gina Giuliano, Kim Stasiak and Cheryl D'Addato, for enduring all of those poses and making the photo shoot run so smoothly.

➡ To Joe Weider, for helping to bring fitness into the mainstream and expanding my knowledge in the early years.

➡ To the numerous professors of nutrition and exercise science who, through your teachings and writings, have furthered my knowledge in a complex field.

➡ To Shonna McCarver, Monica Brant, Susie Curry, Lori Ann Lloyd, Lena Johannesen, Tamilee Webb, Marla Duncan, Amy Fadhli, Lisa Lowe, Donna Richardson, and Amanda Doerrer, for your endorsement of this book. You are true fitness professionals!

➡ To James and Golds Gym in White Plains, NY, for providing me with a fabulous facility to shoot the photos for this book. You guys are the best!

CONTENTS

FOREWORD

Look Great Naked . . .

For me, this phrase has a special meaning. As a professional fitness competitor, my career was always predicated on my appearance. I was constantly being judged on every aspect of my body; its shape, symmetry, hardness, and definition. Consequently, whether I was modeling swimsuits, performing in a fitness show, or making personal appearances, I always had to look my physical best. That is, until late 1997, when, suddenly, my life took a dramatic turn—one that would ultimately change my entire existence.

A couple of months before competing in the 1997 Fitness Olympia, I began to experience sharp pains in my lower back. I knew something was wrong, but I put the discomfort out of my mind. After all, it was my lifelong dream to win the Fitness Olympia—the most prestigious of all fitness competitions—and nothing was going to stop me from achieving my goal. So I continued to train hard and watch my diet, focusing only on the task at hand.

When the big day finally came, I knew I had a great chance to win the show. I performed extremely well in the endurance round, my fitness routine was stellar, and my physique looked as good as it ever had. As the final countdown began, I was cautiously optimistic. Although confident in my appearance, the judging process was so subjective that you never could be sure of the outcome.

"In fourth place," the emcee bellowed, "Susie Curry." My mind was racing—I was still in the running.

"In third place, Lena Johannesen." I breathed a sigh of relief—I had made the top two.

"In second place . . . Saryn Muldrow . . ." Although I had every reason to believe that I had won, it wasn't until the emcee raised my hand and actually declared me the champion that the reality sunk in: I was Ms. Fitness Olympia! Everything that I'd worked so hard to achieve had finally paid off. At that moment, I felt like I was on top of the world.

Unfortunately, my excitement didn't last long. Several weeks after the event, I went to see a doctor about my lower back. His diagnosis caught me completely off guard. It turned out I had a herniated disc in my lower lumbar region, and corrective surgery loomed on the horizon. The news was a total shock. Never in my wildest thoughts did I expect my condition to be so severe. It was then that I realized the inevitable: I would never be able to compete again. This was a huge psychological blow. Fitness and competition had been an integral part of my life ever since I was a kid and, from a mental standpoint, I just wasn't ready to quit.

Soon thereafter, everything started to snowball: I lost my endorsement contracts, requests for seminars dwindled, and calls for photo shoots stopped coming in. My entire life was literally being turned upside down. At first, I felt sorry for myself; then, I became angry. My feelings seesawed between these two emotions, creating a vicious cycle that ultimately led to a deep depression. The adversity simply was too much for me to handle.

Through all this, food became an escape, a means to cope with life's stresses. While I had always strayed a little from my diet immediately after a competition, this time I was completely gluttonous. I started pigging out on anything and everything—bacon cheeseburgers, pizza, ice cream, and French fries—no foods were off limits. On top of that, I had basically become a couch potato. My injury made it difficult to perform many of the activities of daily living. Combined with my depression, I barely had the urge to leave my house. This sedentary lifestyle caused all the excess calories that I was consuming to be stored as fat rather than be burned off for energy.

Denial set in. I knew subconsciously that I was gaining weight, but didn't think it was a big deal. After all, I reasoned, "I'm Carol Semple; I'm a world-class athlete and fitness champion; I can bounce back from anything." So I just kept eating and eating.

Then, one day it hit me: I suddenly realized that none of my clothes fit anymore—my once buffed body had turned soft. At that point I thought, "My gosh, what have I done to myself? How did I allow myself to get so out of shape?" It was kind of ironic because, up until then, I never was able understand how a woman could let herself go. It was doubly unimaginable that it could happen to me. Yet here I was, in the exact same predicament that I used to judge others so harshly.

On the scale I gained about 20 pounds but, in reality, it looked like a lot more. My bodyfat percentage, which was normally around 10 to 12 percent, had ballooned up to 24 percent. Most of the weight had settled in my trouble zones; my hips and thighs were huge; my butt was bigger than ever; even my midsection, which was always one of my best bodyparts, had increased several inches in diameter. And to top it all off, I had lost a good deal of muscle, so my body was loose and flabby, without the firm definition that I had been accustomed to and known for.

Although I could somewhat hide my increased proportions in clothes, rest assured, I wasn't a pretty sight naked! One look in the mirror and I knew I had to get my act together; I needed to take charge of my life again!

Given my personal ordeal with my own particular trouble zones, I'm thrilled to be able to endorse this valuable book. The only way to a great body is through proper exercise and nutrition, and Brad shows you exactly how to go about this difficult task in the most efficient manner possible. Whether you are starting from scratch or are just looking to fine-tune your physique, Brad provides all the information you need to slim down and shape up: The exercise program is beautifully conceived and easy to follow; the nutritional regimen is practical and sensible; and the fat-burning tips are true tricks of the trade that will really help you shed those last few pounds.

Just remember, though, it's one thing to look good in clothes but, as I can attest, quite another to look great naked. Trust me, even fitness models aren't born with great physiques; genetics will take you only so far. It requires diligence, commitment, and determination to conquer your trouble zones—it doesn't happen by wishful thinking. But the beauty is, if you're willing to work for it, you really *can* look great naked. By following the advice in this wonderful book, you'll be well on your way to achieving this goal!

Yours in Fitness and Health,

Carol Semple-Marzetta
1997 Fitness Olympia Champion

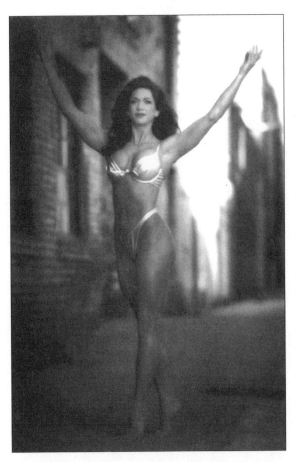

CAROL SEMPLE-MARZETTA
Fitness Angels
c/o Tamarac Athletic
4401 S. Tamarac Pky
Denver CO 80237
303-771-5050
e-mail: bodypatrol@aol.com

INTRODUCTION

Barbara was clearly distressed. "Brad, you need to help me. In two months I'm going to the Bahamas and there's no way I'm putting on a bathing suit looking like *this*!"

Until this time, I had only spoken to Barbara over the phone. Despite her comments to the contrary, she appeared to be in good physical condition. A woman in her early thirties, she was impeccably dressed, wearing a striped business suit hemmed at the knees. Her hair was well coifed and her make-up tastefully applied. Upon casual inspection, I detected no discernible signs of excess bodyfat. "You certainly don't seem to be overweight," I replied. "Specifically what aspect of your body are you unhappy with?"

Barbara blushed for a moment, obviously pleased that her secret wasn't readily apparent. "You really can't tell when I'm wearing clothes," she answered, gently patting her hips, "but, believe me, I need a lot of work before I'll set foot on a beach."

As a personal trainer specializing in women's fitness, I hear this lament on a daily basis. Women are keenly aware of their physical imperfections and become uncomfortable in any situation where they are exposed. In the gym, they'll tie sweatshirts around their waists to cover their butt and thighs. At the beach or pool, they'll pull on a pair of shorts as soon as they have to stand up. While the average guy thinks he's 5 pounds away from being Mr. America, even the skinniest woman thinks she's at least 5 pounds too heavy. In fact, a recent study found that more than 40 percent of women are uncomfortable going nude in front of their own partners!

For many women, clothes can be the great equalizer. Fashion designers are heralded for their ability to develop styles that accentuate the positives and downplay the negatives. By choosing the appropriate cut, color, and pattern, a woman can wear clothes that effectively hide her flaws, presenting her body in the best possible light.

However, to paraphrase Bob Dylan, "At some point, we all have to stand naked." Each morning, a woman has to face herself in the mirror. If she's not happy with what she sees, it is bound to affect her self-esteem, regardless of what others might think.

Fortunately, virtually every woman has the ability to improve her appearance and look great naked—provided she takes the proper approach. By employing the right mix of exercise and nutrition, a great physique can be yours regardless of your present shape.

This book focuses on the trouble zones—the abs, butt, and thighs—and provides all the information that you need to sculpt them to perfection. These are the areas that are most problematic for women—and the areas that are most apparent when you're in the buff. The routine is based on my High-Energy Fitness™ system of training—a supercharged method of exercise that simultaneously tones your muscles while reducing bodyfat. I have spent more than a dozen years perfecting this program with my private clients; it's now available to the general public in the form of this book.

Bodysculpting is at the core of my High-Energy Fitness™ system. Simply stated, bodysculpting is a method of strength training that creates a toned, shapely physique—as opposed to bodybuilding, which focuses more on building big, bulky muscles. Think of each trouble zone as a mound of clay. You are the sculptor—the bodysculptor—and can mold these areas any way you choose. You can add a little here, subtract a little there—do whatever you wish to create the look that you desire. Whether you want to build up, slim down, tighten, or tone, you are in control of your own physical destiny. If you put in the effort, results are guaranteed!

Better yet, the program also is very time efficient. If you're like most women, you are constantly juggling your agenda, trying to fit a myriad of things into a limited amount of time. Job constraints, running a household, raising children—the chores are never ending. With all these responsibilities, you certainly can't afford to spend several hours a day in the gym. The truth is, you don't need to. Each trouble zone requires only about fifteen minutes of training time per session. As you will see, it is the *quality* of training, not the *quantity* of training, that builds a terrific physique. In the case of exercise, less is more. Considering the minimal time commitment, you can't use the excuse that it's impossible to fit a workout into your busy schedule.

I have written this book to be informational, as well as inspirational. Together, we will explore the best way to make your problem areas trouble free and turn your body into a work of art. Here is a preview of what will be covered:

➠ *Chapter 1* discusses the unique problems that women face in their quest to get into shape. In order to develop a great figure, women have to overcome a plethora of physical and mental obstacles. Being aware of these impediments allows you to gain insight into what it takes to conquer these challenges and achieve your body's potential.

➠ *Chapter 2* relates strategies to help you stay motivated in your quest for achieving a better body. The biggest reason that women fail in their fitness endeavors is a lack of dedication. You'll learn specific ways to get into the right frame of mind, set attainable goals, transfer results through visualization, and more.

➠ *Chapter 3* outlines the protocols for the targeted bodysculpting program. No stone is left unturned. Sets, reps, intensity—it's all covered in great detail.

➠ *Chapter 4* delves into the art of exercise performance. As the saying goes, it's not merely what you do, it's how you do it. Here you'll learn how to execute the routine so that results are optimized.

➠ *Chapters 5, 6, and 7* describe targeted training programs for each of the three trouble zones. You'll learn basic muscular anatomy supported by illustrative diagrams that delineate each muscle. Exercises are broken down into groups that target specific areas of your body. A total of 45 different exercises are described in explicit detail. Accompanying the exercise descriptions are photos demonstrating the performance of each move.

➠ *Chapter 8* discusses the fat-burning benefits of cardiovascular exercise. Aerobics complement the targeted bodysculpting workouts, accelerating your ability to get lean and hard. But there's a lot more to aerobics than simply jumping on the bike or treadmill. All the basics are covered: frequency, duration, and intensity. An overview of different cardiovascular modalities is provided, discussing the pros and cons of each.

➠ *Chapter 9* details a complete nutritional regimen to reduce bodyfat and fuel your body. Proper nutrition is vital to achieving a lean, toned physique. Don't think that you can simply exercise your way to a great body—it won't happen. Nutrition is at least as important as exercise in the quest for aesthetic perfection. Many nutritional inaccuracies and untruths are debunked. There are no gimmicks here, only scientifically based concepts that have been proven to work.

➠ *Chapter 10* details expert tips for achieving lasting weight management. These tips are at the cutting-edge of nutrition and are especially applicable for shedding those last few pounds that always seem so hard to lose. By incorporating them into your dietary regimen, you'll turn your body into a fat-burning machine, allowing it to operate at peak efficiency.

➠ *Chapter 11* contains a collection of healthy recipes contributed by some of the top fitness models in the world. These are the favorite recipes of women who make their living by keeping their bodies in top shape. You'll see that eating healthy doesn't have to be boring. Whether it's breakfast, lunch, dinner, or snacks, you'll find delicious recipes that make your mouth water.

➠ *Chapter 12* provides some of my own favorite healthy recipes. Feast and enjoy!

In sum, not every woman can look like a model, or a dancer, or a fitness competitor. Yet every woman *can* maximize her potential and look great naked! By adhering to this program, you will be well on your way to achieving this goal. Never again will buying a swimsuit be as painful as a trip to the dentist. In fact, you'll actually relish the opportunity to try on the teeniest of bikinis. Rather than looking for clothes to camouflage your body, you'll enjoy the freedom to wear whatever you desire—even if it's nothing at all.

A WOMAN'S DILEMMA

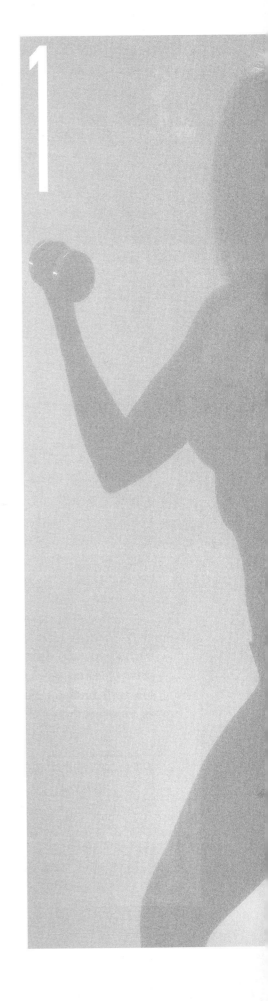

Bodyfat ...

It's unsightly. It's unhealthy. It's unappealing. It's down-
right repulsive. The adjectives are endless. With respect
to the human body, no other word has such a negative
connotation. Its mere mention is enough to make a
woman shudder.

From an aesthetic standpoint, nothing is more
detrimental to your physique than a surplus of bodyfat.
While a certain amount is necessary to pad your internal organs and provide insulation, any excess hangs off
the body like loose jelly, obscuring your muscle tone
and wreaking havoc on your physique.

Women, in particular, are prone to storing bodyfat.
Like it or not, women are the fatter sex; on average, they
carry about double the amount of fat as their male
counterparts. And while men have a propensity to store
fat in their upper bodies, in women it tends to settle in
the dreaded trouble zones: the abs, butt, and thighs.
Hence, as fat accrues, the lower body spreads outwardly,
creating a dumpy, pear-shaped physique. Alas, this is a
woman's dilemma.

Fat Facts

In mammals, fat is contained in cells called *adipocytes*. Adipocytes are pliable store-houses that either shrink or expand to accommodate fatty deposits. They are present in virtually every part of the body. There is a direct correlation between the size of adipocytes and obesity: The larger your adipocytes, the fatter you appear. However, although adipocytes can be reduced in size, they can't be completely expunged. The reality is, once adipocytes form, you are stuck with them for life.

On the surface of each adipocyte are tiny receptors that control the storage and release of fat from the cell. Receptors can be likened to doorways; they either allow fat into or out of adipocytes. There are two basic types of fat receptors: alpha-2 receptors and beta receptors. Taking the doorway analogy a step further, alpha-2 receptors are the "entrances" that let fat into adipocytes for long-term storage, while beta receptors are the "exits" that let fat out of adipocytes to be burned for energy. Depending on various physiologic factors (hormonal stimulus, enzymatic activity, caloric availability, etc.), these receptors ultimately determine whether bodyfat is gained or lost.

The accretion of bodyfat generally begins at the onset of puberty. During this period, there is a surge in the production of estrogen. Estrogen is a hormone that promotes secondary female sex characteristics. Among its many functions, estrogen is integrally involved in the storage of bodyfat. Specifically, it exerts a regional influence on lipoprotein lipase—an enzyme that signals the body to store fat. In lower body adipocytes, estrogen stimulates lipoprotein lipase activity, causing fat to accumulate in this area. Conversely, estrogen has the opposite effect in the upper body, where it actually suppresses the activity of lipoprotein lipase and thereby impedes fat deposition. This site-specific response diverts fat away from the upper body and into the trouble zones, producing the rounded features normally associated with a feminine physique.

When a woman becomes pregnant, bodyfat levels rise even further. Fat is a primary energy source used for fetal development. It helps to nourish the fetus and fuel the growth and maturation of fetal organs, vessels, and bones. In order to support these extra energy requirements, the body attempts to mobilize as much fat as possible. It does so by secreting a large amount of progesterone—a hormone that increases appetite. Progesterone levels remain elevated throughout pregnancy, inducing the intense cravings commonly associated with childbirth. In addition, there is a rapid proliferation of adipocytes. Millions of new fat cells are created, with most of them going directly to the trouble zones. All told, the average postpartum weight gain approaches 30 pounds—much of it in the form of fat.

The aging process also has a negative effect on body composition. Statistics show that the typical woman has approximately 20 percent bodyfat at the age of twenty, 30 percent at the age of thirty, and so on. Thus, by the time a woman reaches her fiftieth birthday, roughly half of her body is comprised of fat. This is largely due to an age-related loss of muscle tissue. Beginning as early as the mid-twenties, women lose roughly 1 percent of their muscle mass each year and continue to do so throughout the rest of their life. Muscle is the most metabolically active tissue in the body; the more you have, the more calories you burn. Thus, a reduction of muscle progressively slows metabolism, causing a gradual but steady increase in bodyfat.

Cellulite

On top of everything, women also have to contend with the big "C": cellulite. It is estimated that up to 90 percent of all women develop some cellulite after the age of thirty. Although these gel-like formations can form anywhere on the body, they are most apt to appear in areas that store the most fat—namely, the dreaded trouble zones.

Cellulite tends to be hereditary; if your mother and siblings are afflicted, the chances are good that you will be too. Like your height, eye color, and hair texture, genetics dictate where fat is deposited and the semblance that it takes on your body. Hence, while some women can be obese with little evidence of cellulite, others can be relatively thin and have cottage cheese thighs. This is simply the luck of the draw. If you picked good parents, you might escape the big "C". If not . . .

To appreciate how cellulite develops, a basic overview of skin composition is in order. The skin and its underlying tissue have three fundamental layers: The top layer is comprised of a cellular-based tissue called the dermis. Its primary purpose is to protect your body from outside contaminants. The middle layer is made up of fibrous connective tissue called superficial fascia. It is substantially thicker than the dermis and acts like an internal stocking to support the skin. The lower layer is made up of adipose tissue—plain old fat. It has several functions including insulating the body, padding the internal organs, and providing a source of long-term energy.

You're probably wondering how all this physiology applies to cellulite. Well, the superficial fascia is responsible for holding bodyfat in place. In men, the superficial fascia is arranged in a criss-cross pattern that is strong and consistent. Accordingly, fat is contained in a uniform manner subcutaneously (below the skin), leaving the skin surface smooth and supple. In women, however, the superficial fascia tends to be irregular and discontinuous. It has a vertical distribution, forming honeycomb-like patterns beneath the dermis. Hence, when fat accumulates, it pushes up toward the skin's surface in clusters, giving the skin the lumpy, dimpled appearance commonly known as cellulite.

Cellulite is further exacerbated by the localized accumulation of lymphatic fluid. Research has shown that cellulite contains an abundance of glycosaminoglycans—a polysaccharide-based compound that has high water-attracting properties. Glycosaminoglycans draw fluid into fatty tissue, causing extensive swelling in cellulite-affected areas. This heightens the density of cellulite, making it heavy and voluminous.

Moreover, because of a decline in the skin's elasticity, cellulite tends to worsen over time. As you age, the skin begins to sag and loses its ability to contain subcutaneous tissue. With its support network diminished, cellulite becomes even more prominent, accentuating the "orange peel" look.

The Skinny on Fat Loss

In order to achieve a lean, defined appearance, bodyfat must be kept to an absolute minimum. This, however, is easier said than done. Americans spend billions of dollars each year in their quest to win the battle of the bulge. Between nutritionists, dieticians, supplements, and the like, the weight loss industry has a higher gross national product than many third world nations! Despite these enormous expenditures, however, more than two-thirds of the population still remains overweight and out of shape.

Weight loss is especially difficult for women. Why is it, I am often asked, that men seem to lose weight rather easily while women struggle to drop a just a few pounds? The answer is related to bodyfat distribution. You see, where you store fat has a direct bearing on how it's metabolized. Research has shown that the lower body has a much greater percentage of alpha-2 receptors than the upper body. As you may recall, alpha-2 receptors are the "entrances" that shuttle fat into adipocytes. With a plethora of fat-hungry alpha-2 receptors, the lower body tends to hoard fat and hold on to it. And since this is the area where women are prone to fat storage, they invariably have a harder time dropping weight.

The rigors of childbirth can make it even more difficult to reduce bodyfat. Throughout term, major biological changes take place. Certain areas expand, others stretch, and still others sag due to the demands of childbearing. Fat cells multiply in abundance. The thyroid gland often becomes sluggish, slowing down metabolism. All in all, the entire body is thrown out of whack. These effects are compounded with multiple pregnancies; after the second or third child, losing postpartum weight becomes even more problematic.

Circulation also plays an important role in fat burning. In order for fat to be metabolized, it must be transported via the bloodstream, where it's shuttled to the liver and other active tissues for use as fuel. Unfortunately, blood flow tends to be poor in fatty areas. While lean muscle has an intricate arteriovenous network, adipose tissue is relatively devoid of these blood vessels. This inhibits the body's ability to harness fat as an energy source, keeping fat-laden regions fat.

Quick Fix Alternatives

In order to combat the battle of the bulge, women are increasingly pursuing alternative courses of action. They'll purchase the newest fitness gizmo, go on the latest fad diet, or even starve themselves to take off weight. It is not uncommon for a woman to be so despondent about her appearance that she resorts to the use of "miracle" pills, creams, and potions as a last-ditch alternative, hoping to find magic in a bottle.

In reality, however, the great majority of weight loss products are little more than glorified snake oil remedies. They are brought to market by unscrupulous hucksters seeking to capitalize on the naivete of the general public. The products have dubious modes of action, with no scientific evidence to support their efficacy.

Making matters worse, the fitness industry is very poorly regulated, giving free reign to a host of unethical marketing scams. As long as a product doesn't allege to treat or cure a disease, it isn't subject to regulation by the Food and Drug Administration. Thus, a company can make exaggerated claims about a product with virtually no fear of reprisal. You've undoubtedly seen or heard some of these outrageous advertisements:

"Lose thirty pounds in thirty days."

"Drop two dress sizes in a week."

"Take it off without even trying."

The ads sound so enticing that you just want to believe them. After all, wouldn't it be great to lose weight without any effort? Unfortunately, there is no such thing as magic in a bottle; if there was, everyone in the world would be buff! Don't be fooled by pie-in-the-sky promises from fly-by-night companies. Ultimately, the only thing you'll end up losing is your money.

There are, however, a few weight loss alternatives that have been accepted into the mainstream. The two that have received the bulk of attention are fat burners and liposuction. Let's discuss each in detail:

➡ ***Fat burners:*** Fat burners are the most popular of all weight loss products. Touted as a quick, easy way to lose weight, they account for about a third of the entire dietary supplement market. Since they are classified as supplements, fat burners can be purchased at virtually any health store or supermarket—no prescription is necessary. In most cases, their primary ingredient is either ephedra or synephrine, exotic herbs that work on your sympathetic nervous system. They function very much like amphetamines, secreting hormones that stimulate your beta receptors to release fat. Frequently, chromium, St. John's wort, guarana, and other ingredients are added to the mix, supposedly heightening results.

There is no doubt that, in the short term, fat burners can be an effective aid in reducing bodyfat. When combined with proper diet and exercise, they do help to jumpstart the metabolism, expediting fat loss.

However, it is important to realize that fat burners are by no means a panacea. Despite their thermogenic (producing body heat) effect, fat burners can only be taken for a few months at a time, making them unsuitable for long-term weight management. Habitual usage leads to a rebound effect that actually inhibits the body's ability to burn fat. Over time, they can cause the beta receptors to become resistant to external stimuli (a phenomenon known as down-regulation).

Ultimately, the beta receptors aren't able to function properly, curtailing the release of fat from adipocytes. Once this happens, bodyfat is bound to return.

Fat burners also aren't without adverse side-effects. Like amphetamines, they have a speedlike effect, producing a buzz that can last for hours. Accordingly, many women experience insomnia, nervousness, and anxiety from their use. More serious ailments, such as seizures and stroke, also have been reported. And because of their tendency to raise blood pressure and heart rate, fat burners are explicitly contraindicated for anyone with hypertension and/or existing cardiac anomalies.

➠ **Liposuction:** Liposuction (lipo, for short) is perhaps the most controversial weight loss option. In just a few short years, lipo has become one of the most commonly performed elective surgeries in the world. Doctors market the procedure as a way to "contour" the body. Just suck out the fat, they assert, and you'll never again have to worry about being overweight. But despite this lofty proclamation, it's really not that cut and dried.

Lipo is a medical procedure performed by a licensed physician. A cylindrical tube is inserted into a fatty area and fat is literally "vacuumed" from the body. It usually is done under local anesthesia on an outpatient basis, making it relatively convenient and safe (although several deaths have been attributed to the procedure usually as a result of the anesthesia).

For the most part, lipo is reasonably effective at removing small amounts of localized fat. The technique has been perfected to the point where there isn't much scarring or discomfort. Recovery is fairly short and, although swelling temporarily obscures results, visible changes can be seen almost immediately.

The trouble is, the effects of liposuction aren't permanent. Regardless of what some physicians would have you believe, without proper exercise and nutrition, bodyfat will return. Excess calories have to be stored somewhere and, rest assured, they'll find their way into fat cells. Areas of the body that never stored much fat will begin to enlarge. The arms, back, neck—places you normally don't associate with fat storage suddenly start to appear pudgy.

And don't think treated areas are immune from regaining weight. Lipo only removes a small percentage of fat cells from a site. There are plenty of existing adipocytes left that are hungry for fat. Once these cells reach a certain size, they undergo a process called hyperplasia, where they divide into more fat cells. That's right, fat cells can regenerate! I've trained many women who've gone through the travails and expense of lipo only to wind up right back where they started.

In the final analysis, neither of these options are appropriate for keeping off bodyfat. Forget about quick fixes; they just don't work. While it's tempting to look for an easy way out, you'll only end up wasting your time and money.

The High-Energy Fitness™ Solution

Fortunately, there is a long-term, permanent solution to a woman's dilemma: High-Energy Fitness™! When combined with proper nutrition, a targeted high-energy routine will help to regulate hormonal response, preserve muscle tissue, and improve vascular circulation—all the ingredients for lasting bodyfat reduction. With dedicated effort, you'll be able to take off weight in all the right places, conquering your trouble zones forever.

And just because you may be predisposed to cellulite doesn't mean you have to succumb to its effects. By reducing bodyfat and adding muscle tone, you can substantially reduce, if not completely eliminate, this unsightly malady. Lean muscle tone helps to smooth underlying fat, making dimples less evident. Once bodyfat is reduced to acceptable levels, your trouble zones will be taut and toned and those lumpy, bumpy mounds of flesh will be a mere memory.

If all this sounds too good to be true, you're in for a pleasant surprise. Thousands of women have successfully used the High-Energy Fitness™ system to redefine their bodies, and so can you. You should start to notice changes within several weeks. You'll feel tighter and firmer, and your clothes will begin to fit better. Soon, others will start to notice these changes, complimenting you on your appearance. Over the next several months, your fat will slowly melt away, and in its place will be lean, hard muscle tone. And before you know it, your body will have transformed before your very eyes!

So put on your sweats, lace up your sneakers, and get ready to forge ahead. A better bod awaits!

STAYING THE COURSE

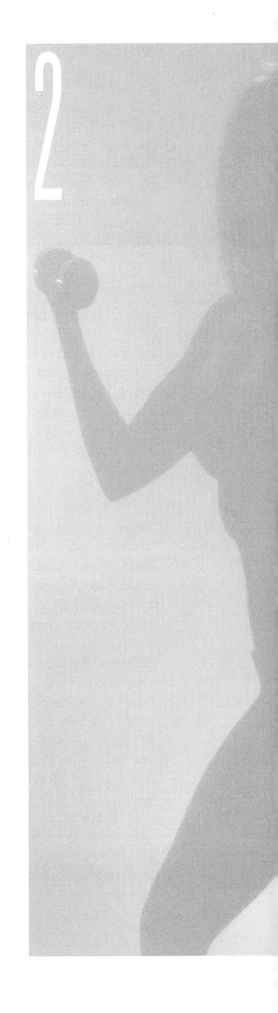

"Everyone keeps telling me how great I look . . . "

While many women cannot envision ever hearing these words, it is a common statement made by those who are determined to maximize their potential. I hear these sentiments regularly from my private clients. One of my biggest joys as a personal trainer is seeing a woman's self-confidence soar to new heights because she has redefined her body.

However, in order to exact a positive change on your physique, you must be driven to succeed. It's not enough to simply want a great bod; you have to make it a priority. Everybody *wants* to look great naked, but few have the determination to make this dream a reality.

Most women start out with the best of intentions and are brimming with enthusiasm when they begin a fitness routine. Initially, they are eager to go to the gym and are committed to attaining their best possible shape. However, within a short period of time, they begin to lose interest in working out. They start to miss workouts and stray from their nutritional regimen. Little by little, their motivation wanes. The sad fact is, after only eight weeks, more than 80 percent end up abandoning their routines.

More than anything else, consistency is the key to achieving results. I can give you the perfect game plan for getting into shape but, if you aren't consistent, you'll never maximize your potential. Once you stop an exercise regimen, all your gains gradually slip away. Your muscles atrophy, your bodyfat returns, and you eventually appear as if you never trained at all.

Fortunately, specific actions can be taken to promote lasting compliance. By following a few basic tenets, you will be compelled to stay on the straight and narrow. Exercise is habit forming and, once a training ritual is established, you'll feel guilty about missing a workout.

Develop a Positive Mindset

With respect to fitness, women often are their own worst enemies. They tend to be self-conscious and insecure about their bodies and perpetually see themselves as being fat and out of shape—regardless of their actual proportions. One of the distinct characteristics of anorexic women is that they are habitually obsessed with being overweight. A 5'8" runway model can look in the mirror and think she's grossly obese. This distorted sense of self-image invariably causes a woman to become despondent and give up on herself, frequently becoming self-destructive in the process.

It therefore is imperative to develop a positive body image. In spite of how you feel about your appearance, always maintain proper perspective. Never put yourself down by saying, "I'm fat" or "I look terrible." These negative thoughts only serve to lower your self-esteem, decreasing your motivation to get into shape. Don't worry about your present condition; you are merely a work in progress. Take solace in the fact that, as long as you maintain a fitness lifestyle, every new day will bring you one step closer to achieving your ideal physique.

Get excited about the fact that you are changing your appearance. Enthusiasm and motivation go hand in hand. As the great poet Ralph Waldo Emerson once said, "Nothing great was ever achieved without enthusiasm." It's amazing how much difference a positive attitude can make in your life. Accordingly, make every effort to avoid negative people. Anyone who tries to bring you down has no place in your life. Heed the old saying: "If you hang around with dogs you get fleas," and associate only with those who are upbeat and share your ideals. I guarantee that it will make a big difference—not only in your physique, but in your everyday life, as well.

Above all, be confident in your abilities. Strike the words "I can't" from your vocabulary. From now on, you must take the approach that you can accomplish anything you set your mind to do. And don't just think it; you must actually believe it. Believing you can do something is half the battle. To paraphrase W. Clement Stone, "Whatever your mind can conceive and believe, you can achieve."

Set Goals

Goals are essential to exercise adherence. If you have a clearly defined purpose to train, you are much more likely to continue, and even look forward to, your workout. Of course, everyone has times when they simply don't feel like training. Sickness, work issues, and other crises can set back your efforts for days or even weeks. However, if you have well-defined goals that are important to you, you will be inclined to get back into your routine in relatively short order.

A goal must be both quantifiable and attainable. If these criteria are not met, the goal is nonspecific and therefore not meaningful. Nonspecific goals cannot be readily achieved and are apt to result in frustration. Let's discuss these criteria in greater detail:

➡ *In order for a goal to be quantifiable, it must have measurable parameters.* For example, losing 20 pounds in three months is a quantifiable goal. You can weigh yourself today and again in three months to see whether you have met your goal. The scale will indicate your degree of weight loss in a measurable context. Other examples of quantifiable goals include reducing your waistline by 3 inches in a month, dropping one dress size in six weeks, etc. Conversely, wanting to look good is not a quantifiable goal. This is subjective and cannot be measured by any defined standards. A "goal" like this is doomed to lead to disappointment and frustration.

➡ *In order for a goal to be attainable, it must be realistic.* For example, losing 20 pounds in three months is an attainable goal. Losing 90 pounds in three months is not. If a goal is not attainable, it can serve as a demotivator. An unattainable goal can make you feel as if your fitness endeavors are pointless. It is better to set modest goals that are readily within reach. This lends to a feeling of accomplishment and spurs you on to loftier goals.

Once you have formulated your goals, break them down into short time frames of no more than three months. By limiting the time horizon of your goals, you are able to accomplish them in a reasonable period of time. This promotes positive feedback and buoys self-confidence. For example, losing 30 pounds might appear to be a daunting task, but losing 6 pounds a month for five months seems eminently more attainable. After a mere thirty days, you can relish the fact that you achieved your goal and set your sights on the next objective.

Whenever possible, create incentives to help you reach your goals. For example, if you want to lose weight, buy an expensive dress that's several sizes too small. The thought of having a beautiful dress sitting unused in your closet should be enough of an impetus to get you in the gym. Alternatively, have your husband or boyfriend agree to take you away on a romantic vacation if you drop a certain number of dress sizes. Getting others involved in your fitness efforts will provide a support network that can spur you on to greater heights. In short, think about out what really motivates you and apply it to what you want to get out of your exercise program. You have to really want something in order to maintain motivation over a period of time. Without a specific goal, you will not have a reason to put in the labor necessary to achieve results. Give yourself an edge and make use of every possible motivator that is meaningful to you—it will inspire you to stay fit for life.

Once you accomplish a goal, you should immediately set a new goal that reflects your mission to work out. This will keep you focused in your efforts and allow you to maintain a high degree of motivation. Review your goals periodically to make sure that they are consistent with your present objectives. Goals will often change as you progress in your fitness endeavors, and reevaluating your position will help to ensure lasting compliance.

Visualize Success

Visualization is a technique that can be used to reinforce your goals and sustain your motivation to train. Essentially, it is an organized form of daydreaming. Many athletes use this technique to actualize their potential. A basketball player, for instance, might visualize swishing a last-second jump shot or a baseball player might visualize hitting a game-winning home run. The technique works beautifully in an exercise setting, where it has been proven to increase adherence and improve training performance.

Visualization is best practiced in a quiet environment without any distractions. It can be done either standing up or lying down. When you are ready, close your eyes and relax your muscles. Begin to think about your physique. Visualize each problem area—your abs, butt, and thighs—and get an image of the way you want them to appear. Think of yourself in great shape, walking on the beach in a bikini, or wearing a sexy dress at an affair. Make the image as clear and realistic as possible, seeing it as a movie on the back of your eyelids.

You might even want to think of a woman whose physique you admire, such as a famous celebrity, fitness model, or perhaps even someone who works out in your gym. Fantasize that you possess the body of your role model and carry this vision into your exercise routine. You may, for example, think of Tina Turner's legs or Demi Moore's abs and picture them on your own body. Let your imagination be your internal source of motivation and, within reason, do not set any boundaries as to what you can accomplish.

Visualization can be enhanced through the use of photos. They say a picture is worth a thousand words. Well, it's also a great means to reinforce a specific mental image. For example, find a picture of yourself when you were happy with they way you looked and tape it to your refrigerator or put it on your dresser. Just make sure that it's in full view. Every time you see this picture it will remind you of your potential and help to keep your image fresh in your mind.

Stay Off the Scale!

"How am I doing?" Ed Koch, the ex-mayor of New York, used to ask this question on a regular basis . . . and so does every woman who begins an exercise program. And who's to blame them? You want to make sure that all your hard work is paying off, right?

For many women, progress is measured in pounds; it all boils down to whether or not they've lost weight. Thus, the good old bathroom scale has become the preferred tool to assess the effectiveness of an exercise program. And the scale has certain benefits. It is convenient and easy to use; just step on the scale and you get an instantaneous readout of your weight.

Be careful, though, that you don't become a slave to the scale. Women tend to be scale-obsessed. They weigh themselves incessantly and freak out as soon as they gain a pound. In this respect, using the scale as a barometer can be deceiving and counterproductive. For instance, the scale does not account for bodyfat percentage or water retention, and thus can give a false impression of actual results. Muscle is much denser than fat and consequently weighs more by volume. A golf ball, for example, weighs more than a tennis ball even though it is much smaller in overall diameter. Similarly, when you adhere to a regimented exercise program, you can actually increase your weight while decreasing your bodyfat percentage. In this way, your weight is "redistributed" and you can reduce your proportions by several dress sizes.

In reality, weight is just a number and means very little in the overall scheme of things. It is much more important to be happy with your shape and like the way that your clothes fit your body. If you choose to weigh yourself, do so no more than once per week. And if you happen to gain a pound or two, take it in stride. As long as you are sticking to this program, positive change will happen—I guarantee it! In the end, defer to the mirror. Let the way you look and feel be the ultimate gauge of your progress.

PROGRAM PROTOCOLS

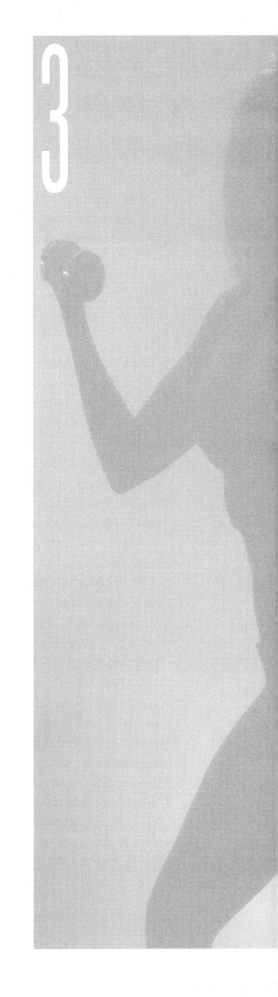

"I've tried everything but I just can't seem to tone up my . . . "

Whether it's the abs, butt, hips, or thighs, women are forever trying to firm their trouble zones. They'll spend hours in the gym, riding, rowing, and stepping their way to what they hope will be a better body. Unfortunately, without a proper course of action, the plight of these women will almost always end in frustration.

There is only one way to get rid of your flab and develop a toned, shapely physique, and that's through a regimented program of exercise and nutrition. Fitness truly is the fountain of youth. It can turn back the clock and reverse the aging process, allowing you to recapture the body you once had. However, simply going to the gym and lifting some weights isn't enough to get the job done. The vast majority of women who undertake an exercise program never see a tangible change in their bodies. The main reason for their failure: lack of knowledge about exercise.

Exercise is a science. Just as you wouldn't attempt to overhaul a car engine without a thorough comprehension of auto mechanics, you can't expect to transform your physique magically without understanding the fundamentals of exercise. Knowledge is power!

Once you've acquired the appropriate knowledge, you are in control of your body and can decide how you want it to look. You can tone, reduce, enlarge, and/or shape your trouble zones to perfection. Within your own genetic potential, there is virtually no limit to what you can achieve.

Fortunately, you don't need to spend countless hours learning the rudiments of exercise physiology. This book provides a foolproof system that takes the guesswork out of training. No stone is left unturned. Everything you need to know is laid out in a structured format, affording you the ability to concentrate on one thing: toning your trouble zones to perfection.

Exercises

All exercises are not alike! It is all too common for a woman to string together a series of exercises fortuitously, neglecting to consider how they interact with each other. The net effect is a hodgepodge of maneuvers that have little cohesion. Ultimately, if you want to rise above the ordinary and look great naked, a more scientific approach is in order.

It is a fact that certain exercises complement one another, working synergistically to produce optimal results. Others merely overlap, providing little additional utility. Unfortunately, even many seasoned fitness professionals do not fully comprehend this reality and continue to train in a haphazard fashion. This misguided approach is not only extremely inefficient, but it actually can decrease performance and compromise results.

In order to simplify the training process, exercises for the various trouble zones have been classified into three groups. Each group contains movements that work your muscles in a specific fashion. By choosing one exercise from each group, you'll optimally target your trouble zones without any wasted effort. All you have to do is mix and match to create a perfect routine every time. It's that easy!

There are five exercises outlined for each group for a total of fifteen exercises per trouble zone: Use them all. Experiment with different combinations and strive to make each workout different from the last. This will help to counteract the adaptation process that takes place from repeatedly performing the same routine on a regular basis. When exercises are overused, your body develops a tolerance to these movements. Ultimately, you reach a training plateau and results stagnate. By employing constant variety, your muscles never can to adapt to a particular exercise. Your workouts will remain a continual challenge and results will proceed at a steady rate.

Reps

Repetitions (reps, for short) are one of the least understood components of exercise. Sure, everyone knows what they are, but few understand their place in a routine. Consider the following: Several years ago, I conducted a survey of prospective clients, asking how many reps they performed in a typical set. The most common answer was "ten." When asked why they chose to train in this rep range, the most common answer was "I don't really know!"

Clearly, the number of reps that you perform shouldn't be a mere afterthought. It is an important training variable that has a profound effect on your physique. To a great extent, it will determine the size and shape of your muscles. Let's discuss the different rep ranges and how they affect your proportions.

➡ ***High reps:*** If you want to improve the definition of a muscle without substantially increasing its bulk, it is best to train in a high-rep range, employing between fifteen and twenty reps per set. High reps target your slow-twitch muscle fibers (also called Type I fibers). These fibers are predominantly utilized during continuous activities sustained for long periods of time. Because of their endurance-oriented nature, slow-twitch fibers have only a limited ability to increase in size. Thus, by targeting these fibers, you'll attain a lean, toned physique with little effect on muscular mass.

In addition, because of the reliance on slow-twitch fibers, high-rep training is a great source for fat burning. Slow-twitch fibers have a large amount of mitochondria—"cellular furnaces" where fat burning takes place—that expedite the use of fat as an energy source. This allows them to get much of their energy by burning fat for fuel. Consequently, training with high reps helps to decrease your bodyfat stores and thereby accentuate lean muscle tone.

➡ ***Moderate reps:*** If you want to increase the size of a muscle, the use of moderate reps is warranted. This entails training with "heavy" weights, using between 6 and 10 reps per set. The goal here is to stimulate your fast-twitch muscle fibers— the ones that have the greatest potential for growth. These fibers (also called Type II fibers) are activated during intense, short-term activities. They are strength oriented and therefore expand in size in order to accommodate the demands of heavy lifting. As a rule, they are the only fibers that have the ability to promote muscular bulk.

However, while moderate reps are great for building muscle, they are a poor choice for burning fat. Moderate reps are decidedly anaerobic; there is very little oxygen expended in performance. Since oxygen is required for the oxidation

Table 2.1 summarizes the effects of training in each rep range.

TABLE 2.1

Rep Range	Number of Reps Per Set	Goals
High	15 to 20	Tone muscle, burn fat
Moderate	6 to 10	Build muscle

of fat, fat burning is abated. Therefore, most of the energy utilized during this type of training is derived from burning glucose, rather than fat, as a fuel source.

It is important to note that, depending on your goals, you can use high reps for one target zone and moderate reps on another. You can, for example, train your glutes with moderate reps to increase their size and train your thighs with high reps to improve their definition or vice versa. Only you can decide what rep range is best for your physique. Assess your trouble zones and select your rep range accordingly.

Regardless of the rep range that you choose, it is imperative to keep your form as strict as possible. Perform each rep in a smooth, controlled manner, without allowing momentum or gravity to dictate your rep speed. If you can't finish your set within the prescribed rep range, the weight is too heavy. Resist the temptation to let your ego get in the way of results, and reduce the amount of weight to a manageable level. This will ensure complete stimulation of your target muscles and decrease the possibility of a training-related injury.

Sets

In most training programs, sets are executed in a straightforward manner. You perform a given number of reps, rest, and then repeat the process several times. However, in order to enhance definition, this program employs a technique called giant sets. A giant set is any set that incorporates three or more different exercises in succession. You move directly from one exercise to the next, without resting in between movements. Hence, you will begin with a Group One exercise, go immediately to a Group Two exercise, and finish by performing a Group Three exercise. All told, you'll perform a total of three giant sets for each trouble zone, taking no more than sixty seconds rest in between each giant set—less, if possible.

During your rest intervals, you will employ a technique called selective muscular stretching. Selective muscular stretching is performed as follows: Upon completion of each giant set, immediately stretch the muscle being trained utilizing the stretching movements discussed next. Try to hold each stretch throughout the entire rest interval and then proceed directly to your next giant set.

Hip and Thigh Stretch ▶

From a standing position, grasp a stationary object such as a pole or exercise machine with your left hand. Bend your right knee and bring your right foot toward your butt. Grasp your right ankle with your right hand and slowly pull your foot upward as high as comfortably possible. Repeat this process on the left.

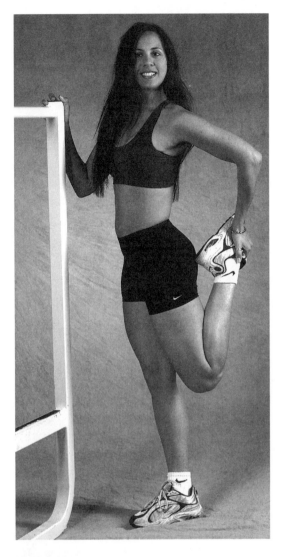

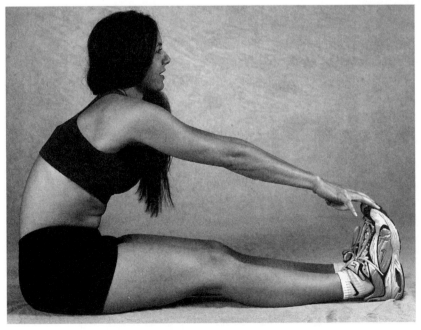

◀ Butt and Hamstring Stretch

From a seated position, straighten your legs and slowly bend forward at the hips. Allow your hands to travel downward along the line of your body as far as comfortably possible. At the point where you feel an intense stretch in your hamstrings, grab onto your legs and hold this position.

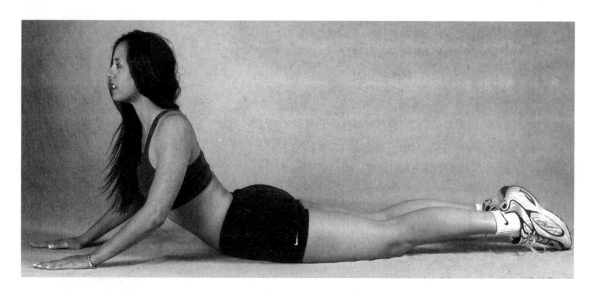

▲   Abdominal Stretch

Lie on your stomach with your palms on the floor. Keeping your legs pressed to the floor, slowly push up with your hands so that your upper body is elevated off the ground and hold this position.

Selective muscular stretching helps to neutralize the effects of lactic acid by restoring blood flow to your working muscles. Lactic acid is responsible for the burning sensation that accompanies intense training and eventually impedes your ability to achieve a muscular contraction. Once it builds up, you simply cannot continue to train. By flushing this byproduct from your body, you are able to regenerate your muscular capacity rapidly, thereby improving performance. Moreover, by expediting nutrient delivery to your musculoskeletal system, selective stretching helps to repair muscle tissue and accelerate the healing process. You experience a diminished amount of delayed-onset muscular soreness and postworkout fatigue. This results in better recuperation between workouts, allowing you to come back strong for your next training session.

Intensity

Of all the training variables, intensity is by far the most important. Simply stated, intensity is the amount of effort expended during exercise. The harder you work, the greater your intensity.

To achieve your full genetic potential, the intensity you apply must be great enough to exceed your body's work threshold—this is called the "overload principle." By nature, the human body strives to maintain a stable state of equilibrium, called homeostasis. If your training intensity doesn't sufficiently tax your resources, there won't be enough of a stimulus to force your body from its homeostatic state. Only by stressing your muscles beyond their physical capacity will they be compelled to produce an adaptive response and exact a change in your body.

For optimal results, you need to train with all-out intensity, taking each set to the point of momentary muscular failure. Weight training is perhaps the only activity where failure is a desired outcome. This is a strange concept for many women to grasp and is often met with a great deal of skepticism. We live in a society where we are rewarded for our accomplishments and punished for our failures. From the time we are born, we are urged to succeed. Failure is always thought of as an unacceptable alternative. However, if you want to look your best, you need to work each muscle to its fullest extent—and that means going all out on each set.

You can't, however, expect to train with all-out intensity from the onset. Your body needs to be acclimated gradually to the effects of intense training. In order to accomplish this task, the routine is divided into three phases: conditioning, developing, and sculpting. Each phase is designed to prepare your body for the succeeding phase. While time intervals are used as a yardstick for progression, don't feel that they are set in stone. Exercise is a very individualized process, and you must progress at your own pace. When in doubt, it is best to err on the side of caution. Don't try to push the envelope. Most women are impatient to see results and prematurely accelerate their training intensity. Resist this temptation. If your body is not yet geared for intense exercise, you invariably will become overtrained and set back your development.

➠ ***Conditioning phase:*** At the onset of training, perform each set at approximately 75 percent of maximum intensity. During this phase, the weights should feel somewhat heavy without causing you to struggle to complete a set. Your goal here is to condition your muscles to the rigors of training and develop the neuromuscular skills necessary for exercise performance. Focus on getting a feel for the routine, concentrating on moving smoothly between movements.

➠ ***Developing phase:*** After three months, your body should be ready for a step-up in intensity. At this point, intensity should be increased to about 90 percent of maximum where the last few reps of a set are a struggle to complete. Your goal here is to develop a tolerance for the discomfort associated with all-out training. Focus on working expeditiously, keeping your heart rate elevated throughout the workout.

➠ ***Sculpting phase:*** After six months, your body should be fully acclimated and ready for all-out training. This means employing 100 percent intensity in your routine, going to physical failure on each set. The last repetition of a set should be extremely difficult, if not impossible, to perform. Make sure that you don't give in to the temporary physical discomfort associated with this type of training. Optimal results can only be achieved by pushing past the pain threshold and taking your body to the limit.

Table 2.2 summarizes the protocols for training intensity.

TABLE 2.2

Stage	Time Frame	Level of Intensity
Beginner/Conditioning	Onset	75%
Intermediate/Developing	Three Months	90%
Advanced/Sculpting	Six Months	100%

Frequency

Contrary to popular belief, exercise doesn't build your muscles—it breaks them down. Intense training places tremendous demands on your body, resulting in a catabolism of muscle tissue, depletion of glycogen reserves, production of free radicals, and fatigue of your entire neuromuscular system. Adaptations to these aftereffects take place in the recovery period, where your body develops muscle tone as a way to cope with future high-intensity stresses. During recovery, your body seeks to repair, replenish, and regenerate itself, becoming harder and more defined in the process.

All too often, women mistakenly subscribe to the theory that if a little bit is good more must be better. They go to the gym and work out on a daily basis, never taking a day off. Don't fall into this trap. By shortchanging recuperation, your body will never have the chance to recover adequately from the extreme demands being placed on it. Inevitably, you will become grossly overtrained and your progress will be brought to a grinding halt. With respect to training, less can be more!

Although women have varying recuperative abilities, you never should train a muscle group on two consecutive days. As a rule, a minimum of 48 to 72 hours is necessary for adequate recovery. Become in tune with your body and know how it responds. If you are feeling fatigued or your muscles are sore, take another day off. When in doubt, it is better to rest a day and come back stronger the next.

Required Equipment

If possible, I recommend that you perform this program in a health club. A good fitness facility will have a vast array of fitness equipment available for use. In the same way that a builder uses a variety of tools to erect a house, a diversity of fitness devices are the "tools" for sculpting your body. While it may be possible for a builder to construct a house using only a hammer and saw, it obviously would be a burdensome task.The end product would be compromised, and the project would take a great deal more time than if he had a full compliment of power tools at his disposal. Similarly, if your access to fitness equipment is restricted, there will be limitations as to the possibilities for your routine. Inevitably, this will serve to delay or restrain your progress.

However, for some women, financial and/or logistical concerns prevent them from training in a gym. If this is your predicament, don't fret. The program is perfectly suited to be performed at home. Although you'll be slightly limited in your choice of exercises, there still are plenty of options to create a varied routine. Accordingly, where applicable, I have provided alternate home-based movements for many of the gym-based exercises. If you opt to go it at home, you will need the following equipment:

⇒ *Dumbbells:* Dumbbells are an essential component of any home gym. You probably will need a set of 2-, 3-, 5-, 8-, 10-, 12-, 15-, and 20-pound dumbbells. Depending on your strength levels, additional dumbbells might be necessary.

⇒ *Ankle Weights:* Ankle weights provide increased resistance for bodyweight movements. Get ones that can accommodate 10-pound weight insertions. Depending on your strength levels, a second set may be necessary.

⇒ *Elastic Strength Bands:* Strength bands simulate cable exercise movements. Because they have a unique strength curve, they are an excellent complement to free weight exercises.

⇒ *Bench:* Although not an absolute necessity, it is advisable to buy an adjustable weight bench. This will allow you to train at an incline, affording the ability to vary your movements and hit your muscles from different angles.

Isotension

As an adjunct to your training routine, you should employ a technique called isotension. To many, this probably sounds like a clinical term for a new form of stress management. However, utilizing isotension can dramatically increase your muscle tone, producing the hard, defined look that women covet.

Isotension, simply stated, is the contraction of a muscle without the use of an external weight. For instance, if you flex your arm so that your biceps enlarges and hold this position, you are utilizing isotension. The same principle can be applied to your trouble zones. For instance, to harden your midsection, simply truncate your abdominals so that they squeeze together. As you contract, feel the abs getting hard and tight. Hold this contraction for about thirty seconds and then relax. After a short rest of no more than fifteen seconds, repeat the process. Spend five minutes or so using the technique on your trouble zones after each workout; it won't take long to see results.

Other Muscle Groups

Although this program focuses on adding shape and definition to your trouble zones, I strongly urge you to train the rest of your body at least once per week. Your muscles function holistically, working together in an agonist/antagonist fashion. When one muscle contracts, its antagonist lengthens, creating smooth, controlled movement. Thus, neglecting areas of your body can lead to structural imbalances between muscle groups. Not only does this ruin the symmetry of your physique, but it substantially heightens the prospect of injury.

Moreover, as previously discussed, muscle tissue is metabolically active. For each pound of muscle that you add, you increase your body's fat-burning potential by fifty calories a day. If you only train your trouble zones and neglect the other muscle groups, more than half of your body's muscle-building capacity is bypassed.

For specific routines and exercises, consult my book *Sculpting Her Body Perfect* (Human Kinetics, 800-747-4457). It outlines a total-body approach to achieving your ultimate body.

THE ART OF PERFORMANCE

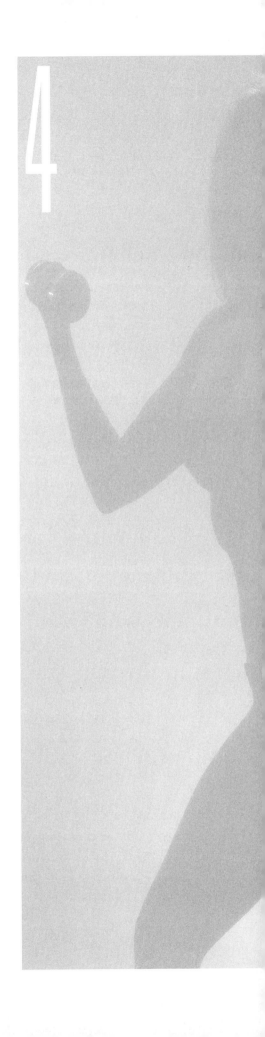

In the preceding chapter, you learned the basic protocols for targeting and toning your trouble zones to perfection. By following these protocols, you will be well on your way to looking great naked. However, having a terrific training routine is only part of the equation. Exercise is more than just information; it also requires implementation. Without a clear grasp of proper exercise performance, you won't be able to put the protocols into practice. Ultimately, your results will be compromised and you'll fall short of reaching your potential.

It is amazing how few people actually know the correct way to exercise. Whenever I walk into a gym, I see the same training mistakes being made over and over. Sloppy form, incorrect breathing, momentum-driven repetitions—the list goes on. At best, these individuals reap only minimal rewards from their efforts; at worst, they end up suffering a debilitating injury. And being an experienced trainee doesn't ensure proper performance; many of the worst offenders have been exercising for years.

It really doesn't take much to become skilled in the fine points of exercise performance. By simply paying heed to a few key training principles, you'll be far ahead of the masses. It will take a little time before you are able to integrate these principles in a seamless fashion. But with consistent practice, you'll soon have a firm grasp of proper lifting technique.

Perfect Form

Perfect form. Everyone wants it; few have it. Whether it's the sweet swing of a professional golfer or the effortless grace of an Olympic skater, perfect form is a thing of beauty.

In the context of weight training, perfect form involves performing an exercise so that only the target muscles are used to complete the maneuver. There are no extraneous body movements; the weight is lifted in the most efficient manner possible, allowing the muscle to contract directly in line with its fibers. No hesitations. No jerky, bouncing movements. Just one continuous motion, with each rep flowing smoothly into the next.

Unfortunately, most women learn how to train through trial and error. They'll watch a fitness show on cable TV or read a magazine and somehow believe they know how to train. Virtually no effort is made to learn exercise fundamentals. The end result can be frightening. Movements are performed in a fashion that bears little resemblance to the way they're supposed to look. And, since they don't realize that their technique is amiss, these women continually make the same mistakes time and again.

Perfect form doesn't come naturally. Even if you're athletically inclined, you can't expect to walk into a gym and breeze through your workout. The human body always tries to take the path of least resistance. It automatically attempts to lift a weight in the easiest possible fashion—not in a way that maximizes muscle tone. Thus, without a clear grasp of proper technique, your secondary muscles will take stress away from your target muscles. Ultimately, structural imbalances are created, resulting in disproportionate development of your physique. Worse, your joints become unduly stressed during exercise performance, heightening the possibility of sustaining a training-related injury.

I have furnished detailed descriptions for every exercise in this book. Make an effort to commit them to your subconscious. But don't simply memorize these movements; understand their function. Know the purpose of each exercise and be aware of the specific muscles that are activated in their performance. As you progress, try to gain insight into the subtleties of exercise biomechanics. The fact is, even minor adjustments in technique can make a big difference in your results.

EXPERT TIP

Always train a muscle over its full range of motion. This allows you to achieve more forceful muscular contractions. There is a direct correlation between the amount of applied force and muscular development; the greater the force, the better your development. Hence, only by working a muscle over its full range will optimal results be attained.

Remember the ABCs

The subject of rep speed has been a source of great debate among fitness professionals. On one end of the spectrum are those who advocate the use of super-slow reps. They feel that weights should be lifted at a virtual snails pace, taking up to fifteen seconds to perform a rep. On the other end of the spectrum are the speed-rep proponents. They believe in training explosively, performing reps in rapid succession. So who's right? In truth, while both of these theories have certain benefits, neither is very practical from a body sculpting perspective. Clearly, for the woman who wants to look great naked, a middle ground is more appropriate.

With respect to rep speed, remember the ABCs of lifting—Always Be in Control. It is relatively unimportant how fast a repetition is performed, as long as the weight remains under control throughout the exercise (unless you are trying to improve speed strength, in which case explosive movements are beneficial). Control is directly influenced by gravitational force, which, in turn, is dictated by the two phases of a repetition (concentric reps and eccentric reps).

Concentric reps (sometimes called positives) involve lifting a weight against the force of gravity. For example, in the hanging knee raise (see page 45), this involves bringing your legs from a position of perpendicular to parallel with the floor. During the concentric phase, you shorten the target muscle until a complete contraction is achieved at the top of the movement. Here, significant exertion is required to complete the lift. Because of the effort involved, a slightly faster pace is acceptable; take approximately two seconds to complete this phase.

Alternatively, eccentric reps (sometimes called negatives) move with the force of gravity. In the example of the hanging leg raise, this involves bringing your legs from parallel back down to a perpendicular position. During the eccentric phase, the muscle is lengthened and stretched at the end of the movement. Your focus here should be on resisting the pull of gravity so that momentum does not take over in performance. On average, the negative phase should last twice as long as the positive, taking about four seconds to complete.

Finally, avoid the tendency to speed up as you approach the end of a set. The last few reps are always the most challenging. Not only are you fatigued, but your muscles experience the intense burn associated with lactic acid buildup. At this point, it's only natural to try to get the set over with as fast as possible. Don't give in to this temptation! Instead, become oblivious to the discomfort and maintain a steady pace. The pain is only temporary; the payoff is well worth it!

EXPERT TIP

Try to maintain a rhythm as you train. Rhythm is an essential part of exercise. It helps you establish a training groove, keeping your concentration on the task at hand. Once a pulse is established, you will settle into a comfortable training pace. As long as you are in a controlled rhythm, your rep speed will take care of itself.

Don't Hold Your Breath

What can be more natural than breathing? Breathing is the essence of life—a basic function that is inbred from the time you are born. You don't need to think about taking a breath—you just do it.

Yet, during weight training, breathing becomes complicated. Rather than breathing naturally, you must inhale and exhale in sync with each repetition—a process that requires conscious thought. This often causes a woman to become discombobulated and lose focus. It's hard enough just struggling to perform an intense set with perfect form; having to remember when to breathe only serves to confuse the situation. Fortunately, within a short period of time, proper breathing becomes second nature.

You must, however, make sure to learn correct technique from the onset; once you fall into bad habits, they can be hard to break. For best results, breathing should be regimented in the following manner: Begin by taking a deep breath before commencing your set. As you initiate the concentric portion of the rep, start to exhale, expelling your breath in an even manner. By the time you contract your target muscle, all of the air should be fully released from your lungs. Then, on the eccentric portion of the movement, inhale as you return the weight to the start position, preparing yourself for the next repetition. Continue breathing in this fashion until your set is completed.

Under no circumstances should you ever hold your breath while lifting (a phenomenon known as the *Valsava maneuver*). Doing so causes a dramatic increase in intra-abdominal blood pressure, which cuts off the blood supply to your brain. Complications such as headaches, dizziness, and fainting are apt to occur. In extreme cases, you can even rupture a blood vessel or tear a retina. Needless to say, the consequences can be dire. The bottom line: Even if you breathe incorrectly, it is better than not breathing at all.

EXPERT TIP

A good way to regulate breathing patterns is to count your reps out loud. On each repetition, count in deliberate fashion: wo-one, two-oo, three-ee, etc. Make sure that you actually say the words; don't just mouth them. This will ensure that air passes through your vocal chords and is expelled on the contraction. As long as you continue counting, it's impossible to miss a breath! Moreover, you don't need to think about breathing properly, freeing your mind to focus on the set.

Mind in Muscle

Mind in muscle ...

To most, this sounds like a contradiction in terms. After all, muscle is normally associated with feats of strength, not acts of intellect. Similarly, there is a prevailing misconception that weight training is merely the action of lifting a weight from point A to point B. All too often, women think that by mindlessly performing a few sets of an exercise, they'll magically transform their physique into a work of art. Sadly, those who subscribe to this theory are doomed to fall short of their aspirations.

Contrary to popular belief, lifting weights is more than just a physical endeavor. Your mind plays an important role in the development of your physique and, in order to maximize gains, it is essential to harness your mental acuity. In fact, two women using identical exercise routines will achieve vastly different results depending on their mental approach to training. There is no doubt: If you want to look great naked, it is essential to use your mind, as well as your body, during your workout.

In order to get the most out of your efforts, you need to develop a mind-to-muscle connection. Simply stated, a mind-to-muscle connection is the melding of mind and muscle so that they become one. It entails visualizing the muscle you are training and feeling that muscle work throughout each repetition. Rather than thinking about where you feel a muscular stimulus, you must think about where you are *supposed* to feel the stimulus. While this concept may seem ethereal at first, in short order, its benefits will become readily apparent.

Establishing a mind-to-muscle connection is beneficial on two levels. First, it ensures that your target muscles perform the majority of work during an exercise. Otherwise, your supporting muscles and connective tissue tend to dominate the lift, diminishing your results. Second, it forces you to utilize proper exercise form continually. When you are mentally locked into a movement, your biomechanics automatically fall into place. This not only helps to improve exercise performance, but it substantially reduces the possibility of a training-related injury.

Developing a mind-to-muscle connection requires consistent practice. From the moment you begin a set, your thoughts must be fixated on the muscle that you are training. You must be oblivious to your surroundings, with all outside distractions purged from your mind. Forget about your nail appointment, your dinner reservations, or any other diversions that might arise. The only thing that matters at this point is the task at hand: sculpting your target muscles to perfection. As you train, make a concerted effort to visualize your target muscles doing the work, without assistance from supporting muscles. When you reach the contracted phase of the movement, consciously feel the squeeze in your target muscles. And, on the negative, feel your target muscle lengthening as you return to the start position. Throughout each set, make this practice a ritual. In short order, it will become habit.

Don't be discouraged if it takes longer to develop a mental link with certain muscles than with others. Generally speaking, it is easier to connect mentally with the muscles of your arms and legs than it is with those of your torso. However, with dedication and patience, you soon will be able to connect with all the muscles in your body, paving the way to better development.

EXPERT TIP

Your mind-to-muscle connection can be enhanced through the use of a technique called guided imagery. Guided imagery is an extension of visualization (discussed in Chapter 2). With this technique, you visualize the way you want your muscles to look and then imagine them taking this form as you are training. For instance, when working your abs, envision yourself with a well-defined six pack, devoid of any bodyfat. As you perform a set of crunches, think of your midsection becoming tighter and harder. Make the image as vivid as possible. With each repetition, see yourself getting one step closer to achieving your ultimate goal. By tapping into the power of your subconscious mind, you can take your body to new heights, turning fantasy into reality.

SEXY ABS

The abdominals can be one of the sexiest parts of the female physique. They are the centerpiece of your body and help to delineate your overall shape. A small waist and flat tummy project a tapered appearance, depicting the classic hourglass figure. If you want to look great naked, six-pack abs are an absolute must.

But you don't have to be naked to enjoy the benefits of a well-defined stomach. There are a plethora of midriff-baring clothes specifically designed for those with abs of steel. Crop tops, belly shirts, and sports bras can be chic and seductive—if your middle is up to the task.

Regrettably, for most women, achieving a tight, toned midsection is a never-ending struggle. Some train for hours on end without seeing tangible results. Due to the physiologic effects of menstruation, toning the lower abdomen tends to be especially problematic. As every woman is well aware, monthly bloating swells the pelvic region. The body adapts to this response by outwardly stretching the pelvic muscle. For those who have endured pregnancy, the muscle is stretched even further. Over time, this causes the lower abs to become soft and pliable, resulting in a distinct pelvic bulge.

To make matters worse, women often have a layer of fat obscuring their abs. Along with the thighs, the stomach is one of the first places where bodyfat is stored. Thus, when excess calories are consumed, a "spare tire" manifests, concealing any hint of muscle tone.

Unfortunately, abdominal training will not eliminate fat deposits in your midsection. You can crunch until the cows come home, but it simply won't decrease the size of your stomach. Despite the outlandish claims by companies that make the "gut-blasters" seen on late-night infomercials, you cannot spot reduce fat—it is a physiologic impossibility. The fact is, if a layer of fat surrounds your middle, all of your hard work in the gym will go unnoticed.

There are three basic factors that will help you lose your belly: strength training (which increases resting metabolic rate), regular cardiovascular exercise (which burns calories), and proper nutrition. Combining these elements into a cohesive fitness regimen will gradually strip away excess adipose, revealing your hard-earned muscle. If you work hard and eat smart, results are sure to follow.

With that said, targeted abdominal training is the key to attaining a rock-hard midsection—one that truly looks great naked. By strengthening your abs, you create an anatomic girdle that prevents your internal organs from protruding outward and counteracts the effects of monthly bloating. Ultimately, this stabilizes your abdominal wall, giving your stomach a flatter appearance. Moreover, by bringing out muscular detail in your midsection, you develop the coveted "six pack" that epitomizes a fit physique. With consistent effort, you'll sport a washboard stomach that looks great—whether or not you're wearing clothes.

However, to train your abs effectively, it is essential to minimize hip flexor involvement. As the name implies, the hip flexors are a group of muscles that assist in flexing your hip. They come into play whenever you bend forward at the waist or lift your legs upward. While strengthening these muscles is important for overall fitness, their influence during ab training can seriously compromise your results. Since the hip flexors are much stronger than the abs, they tend to dominate in exercise performance. When this occurs, your abs are hardly working at all. The net effect: poor abdominal development.

All the exercises that follow have been carefully chosen to diminish hip flexor activation. Movements such as the sit-up, which incorporate excessive bending at the waist, are explicitly avoided. The intent is to maintain constant tension on your abs, working them from multiple angles with a variety of different movements. Ultimately, this ensures complete stimulation of your entire abdominal complex.

A final note: It somehow has been taken as gospel that the abs can and should be trained daily to reap maximal rewards. Even many seasoned fitness professionals still subscribe to this misguided perception. However, this goes against the principles of exercise science. As previously discussed, muscle tissue is actually broken down during exercise—not built up. It is during rest when your body begins to repair this damaged tissue, fueling the acquisition of muscle tone. Short-circuiting the recuperative process doesn't allow adequate time for your abdominal muscles to regenerate, ultimately impeding your progress.

Moreover, your abs are worked indirectly while training other muscle groups. If you train with weights on a consistent basis, your abs get ancillary stress every time you work out—a detail often overlooked when designing a routine. Exercises such as triceps pressdowns, squats, and others all utilize abdominal assistance in their performance. Consequently, the frequency with which you train your abs must be mitigated based on these factors. As with any other muscle group, a minimum of 48 hours is needed between training sessions.

Anatomy of the Abs

The abdominal complex is made up of four distinct muscles: the rectus abdominis, external obliques, internal obliques, and transverse abdominis. Let's take a look at the form and function of each muscle:

➡ The **rectus abdominis** is one long sheath of muscle that runs from just underneath the breastbone (sternum) all the way down into the pelvis. There is a prevailing misconception that the upper and lower portions of the rectus abdominis are two separate muscles that can be trained independently of one another; this is not the case. Due to its configuration, the entire complex contracts as a single unit. Consequently, you cannot work one part without affecting the rest of the muscle. However, by altering the point where spinal movement occurs, it is possible to accentuate one aspect more than another.

➡ The obliques consist of two separate muscles: the **external obliques** and the **internal obliques**. These are the so-called waist muscles that run diagonally along the sides of your body. When properly developed, they give your waist a sleek, tapered appearance. The external obliques are the more visible of the two muscles, spanning from the upper part of your ribs all the way down to your hips. The internal obliques lie underneath the external obliques and thus are somewhat hidden from view. For the most part, both muscles work together as a unit, helping to bend or twist your torso sideways.

➡ The **transversus abdominis** lies deep within your abdomen. Although it is not outwardly visible on the body, the transversus abdominis plays a central role in containing your internal organs as well as assisting in pulmonary function. Due to its position, direct stress really cannot be applied to this muscle. It does, however, act as a stabilizer in the performance of many abdominal exercises and thus receives considerable ancillary stress during training.

Figure 5.1 provides an anatomic diagram that delineates the location of the abdominal muscles.

FIGURE 5.1

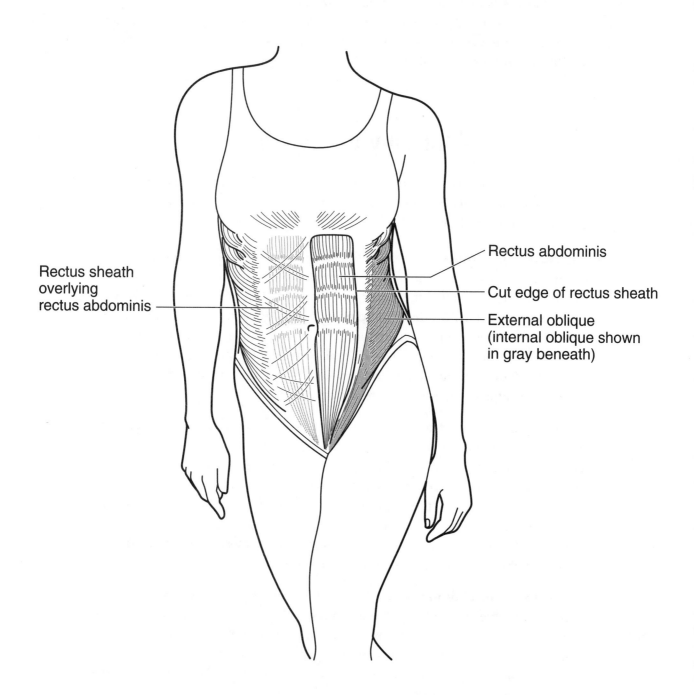

Rectus sheath overlying rectus abdominis

Rectus abdominis

Cut edge of rectus sheath

External oblique (internal oblique shown in gray beneath)

Abdominal "Dos and Don'ts"

The following are common mistakes made during abdominal training that should be explicitly avoided.

➡ ***Don't*** *hold your breath:* While breathing is an integral part of exercise performance, it is especially important during abdominal training. By holding your breath when performing an abdominal movement, your intra-abdominal pressure increases dramatically. This causes your spine to become rigid, diminishing your ability to achieve a muscular contraction.

➡ ***Do*** exhale on the positive portion of the rep and inhale on the negative. If you have difficulty remembering to breathe, count your reps out loud. This will force air to be expelled on each rep.

➡ ***Don't*** *place your hands behind your head:* All too often, women clasp their hands behind their head during abdominal training. Inexplicably, many fitness professionals continue to teach this hazardous practice. However, when your abdominal muscles become fatigued, there is a tendency to pull your neck forward during performance. This puts a great deal of stress on the cervical vertebrae and can lead to serious injury.

➡ ***Do*** keep your hands folded across your chest or rest them at your ears. This ensures that your abs do all the work during exercise performance.

➡ ***Don't*** *use momentum:* Many times, women swing their legs or jerk their torso in an effort to complete a rep. They bounce up and down like a jack-in-the-box, trying to pump out as many reps as possible. However, since your lower back works antagonistically with your abs, it is extremely vulnerable to any sharp movements. Improper abdominal training is a frequent cause of lower back injury.

➡ ***Do*** focus on achieving quality repetitions. It's no big deal if you are unable to reach your target rep range. Over time, your endurance will improve and the amount of reps that you can perform will increase.

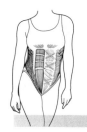

ABDOMINAL exercises

Group One

Group One exercises target the upper abdominal region. For most women, the upper abs tend to develop rather easily. Because the muscle in this area is quite dense, it responds well to intense exercise. On average, you should begin to notice upper abdominal definition within a few weeks of undertaking this training program—provided you don't have a significant amount of bodyfat.

The upper abs receive maximal stress during movements that flex your spine from the upper torso. Focus on rolling your upper body forward as far as possible, bringing your head and chest down toward your hips. In order to limit hip flexor involvement, your lower back must remain completely stable throughout the move. Your torso should only move about 30 degrees in total—any further, and your hip flexors will begin to kick in. While this might seem like a shortened repetition, it's all that is needed to achieve a full muscular contraction.

Group 1

CRUNCH (page, 37)

LYING MACHINE CRUNCH (page, 38)

KNEELING ROPE CRUNCH (page, 39)

SEATED MACHINE CURL (page, 40)

TOE TOUCH (page, 41)

ABDOMINAL exercises

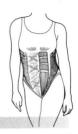

CRUNCH

Begin by lying face up on the floor with your feet planted firmly on the floor. Keep your thighs perpendicular to the ground and your hands folded across your chest. Slowly raise your shoulders up and forward toward your chest, shortening the distance of your trunk. Feel a contraction in your abdominal muscles and then slowly reverse direction, returning to the start position.

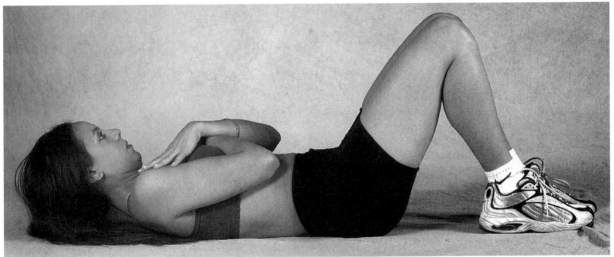

start

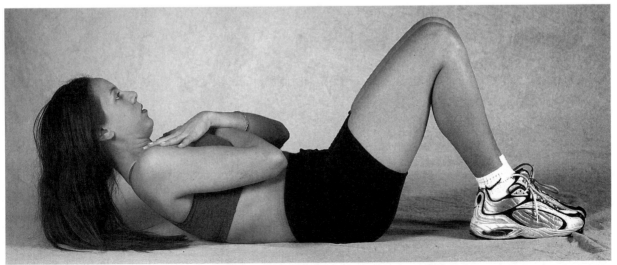

finish

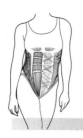

LYING MACHINE CRUNCH

Begin by lying face up in a crunch machine with your feet hooked underneath the restraint pads. Keep your thighs perpendicular to the ground and your hands folded across your chest. Slowly raise your shoulders up and forward toward your chest, shortening the distance of your trunk. Feel a contraction in the your abdominal muscles and then slowly reverse direction, returning to the start position.

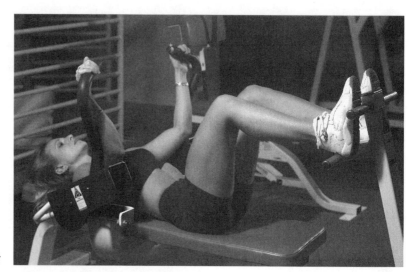

start

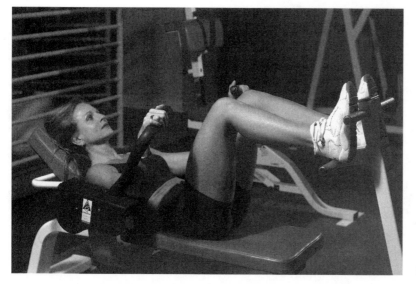

finish

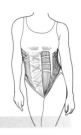

KNEELING ROPE CRUNCH

Begin by kneeling in front of a high pulley apparatus with your body facing the machine. Grasp a rope attached to the pulley and keep your elbows in toward your ears. Slowly curl your body downward, bringing your elbows to your knees. Contract your abs and then slowly uncurl your body, returning to the start position.

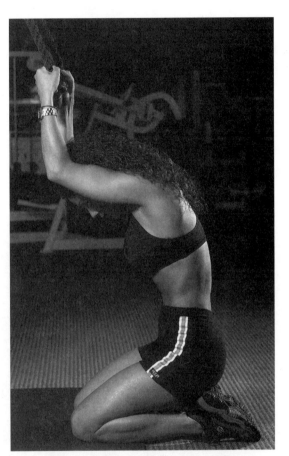

start

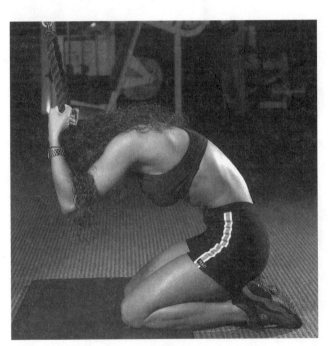

finish

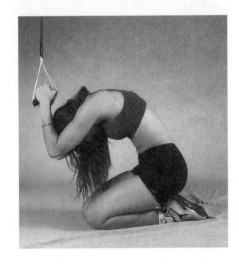

For Home Use: Place a strength band over a door or secure overhead bar (such as a chinning bar) and perform move as prescribed. ▶

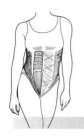

ABDOMINAL exercises

SEATED MACHINE CURL

Begin by sitting in the unit, adjusting the seat so that the pad rests across your chest. Holding onto the pads for support, slowly curl your torso forward, bringing your chest down toward the floor. In order to prevent your hip flexors from taking over, flex only from your upper spine and keep your lower back stable. Feel a contraction in your abs and then return to the start position.

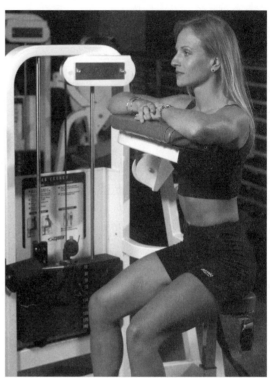

start

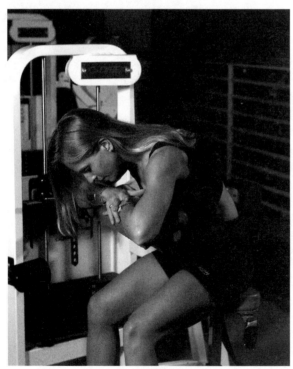

finish

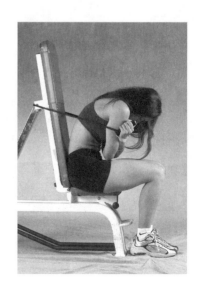

For Home Use: Sit in a chair and wrap an elastic band around the chair back. Cross your arms in front of your chest, holding one end of the band in each hand. Perform the move as prescribed. ▶

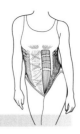

ABDOMINAL exercises

TOE TOUCH

Begin by lying flat on the floor with arms and legs straight up, perpendicular to your body. Slowly curl your torso up and foward, raising your hands as close to your toes as possible. Contract your abs and then reverse direction, returning to the starting position.

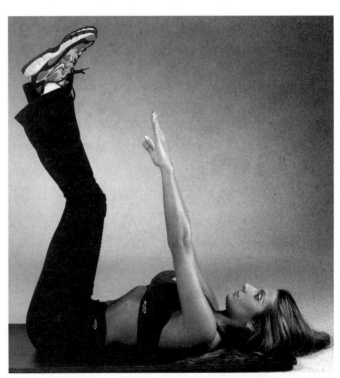

start

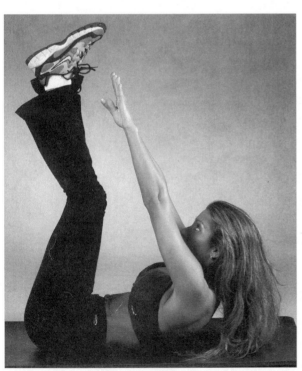

finish

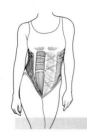

Group Two

Group Two exercises target the lower abdominal region. As previously discussed, physiologic factors make it arduous for many women to achieve lower abdominal definition. To further complicate the situation, this area is especially hard to train. As opposed to the upper abs, there isn't a great deal of pelvic muscle. The rectus abdominis tapers down in width and thickness, leaving only a thin sheath below the level of the navel. As a result, you really don't have a lot of muscle to work with. Moreover, since the pelvis has a limited range of motion, it is difficult to contract the lower abs forcefully.

Despite these obstacles, targeted training can tone your pelvic region and give your lower abs a firm appearance. Don't, however, expect it to be easy. Due to the structural weakness of the lower abs, other muscles will dominate in exercise performance unless you pay strict attention to proper form. You must concentrate on raising your pelvis up toward your stomach, forcing your lower abs to contract. Make sure that your pelvis initiates the move—not your legs. Otherwise, your hip flexors will be doing all the work.

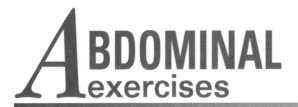 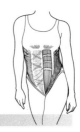

ABDOMINAL exercises

PELVIC TILT

Begin by lying on your back with your knees bent. Keep your feet flat on floor and your arms at sides. Press the small of your back against the floor, flattening your spine until there is no curvature to your lower lumbar region. Your hips will tilt upward as you execute the move. Contract your abs and then reverse direction, returning to the starting position.

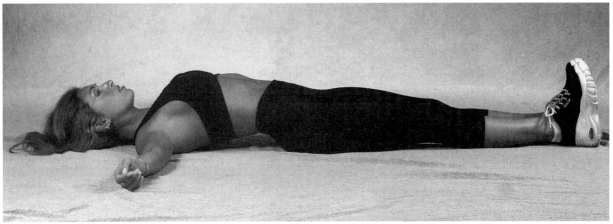

start

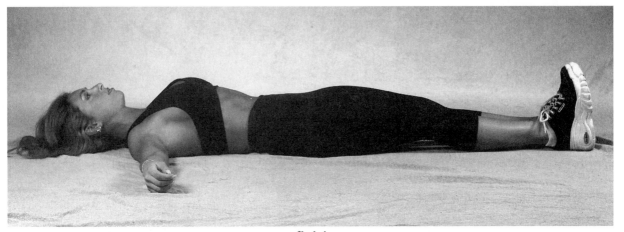

finish

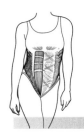

REVERSE CURL

Begin by lying back on the floor. With your hands at your sides, raise your butt as high as possible while keeping your upper back pressed to the floor. Contract your abs and then reverse direction, returning to the starting position.

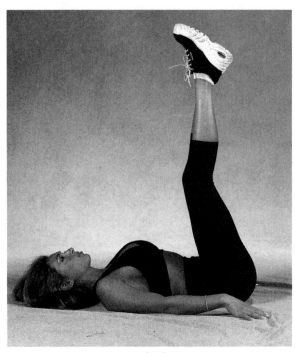

start

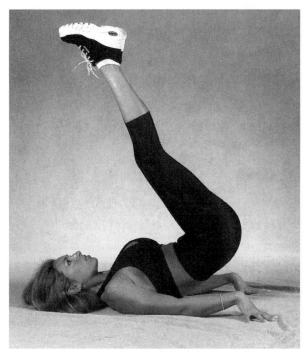

finish

ABDOMINAL exercises

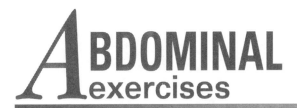
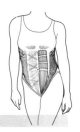

HANGING KNEE RAISE

Begin by grasping a chinning bar with a shoulder-width grip and keep your upper torso motionless throughout the move. Keeping your knees bent, slowly raise your legs upward, lifting your butt so that your pelvis tilts toward your stomach. Contract your abs and then reverse direction, returning your legs back to the start position. For increased intensity, straighten your legs while performing the move.

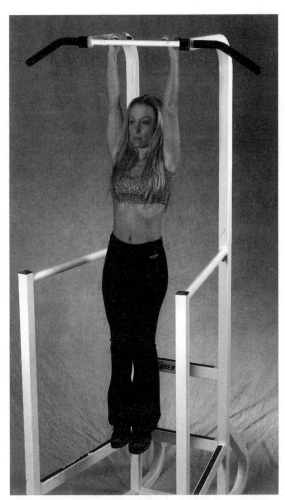

start

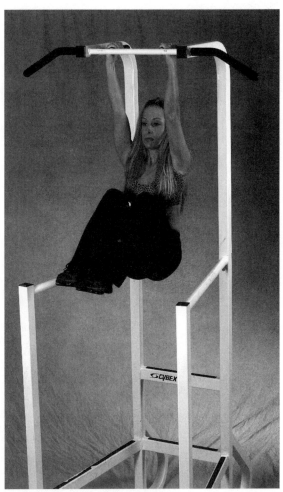

finish

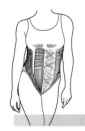

PEDALING

Begin by lying back on a flat bench with your legs straight out and slightly elevated off the bench. Holding on to both sides of the bench, slowly bring your right knee towards your torso, lifting your right glute off the bench in the process. As you return your right leg to the start position, bring your left leg toward your torso in the same manner. Continue this movement, alternating between right and left legs as if pedaling a bike.

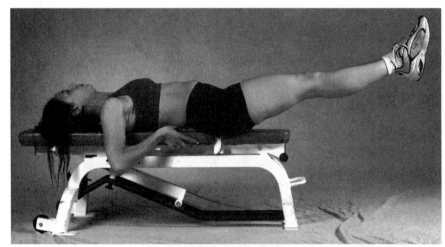

start

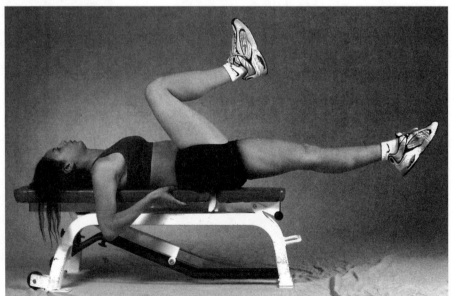

finish

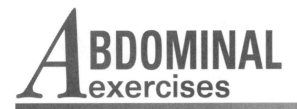

ABDOMINAL exercises

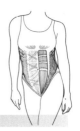

ALTERNATING HANGING KNEE RAISE

Begin by grasping a chinning bar with a shoulder-width grip and keep your upper torso motionless throughout the move. Slowly raise your right knee up and in, lifting your butt so that your pelvis tilts toward your stomach. Contract your abs and then reverse direction, returning to the start position. Repeat this process with your left leg and then alternate between sides until the desired number of reps has been reached.

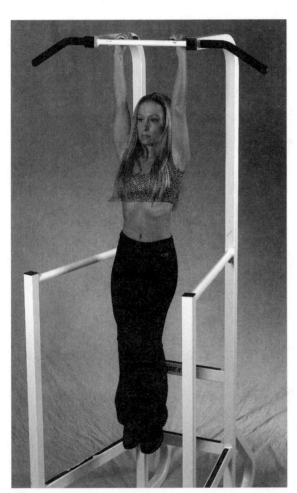

start

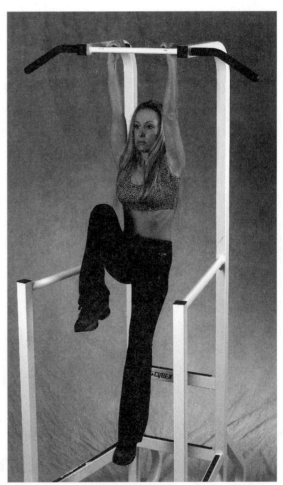

finish

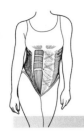

ABDOMINAL exercises

Group Three

Group Three exercises target the internal and external obliques. When properly developed, the obliques provide the finishing touches to your midsection, giving your body a polished look. Say goodbye to those love handles—firming your obliques will keep your waist looking fit and trim.

The obliques are stressed during spinal rotation and lateral flexion—movements that require twisting or bending your body to the right or left. These movements can originate either from the upper or lower body, using modifications of the crunch and leg raise or unique actions specific to the obliques.

A word of caution: The use of weighted movements generally is not recommended when working your obliques. Moves like weighted side bends or weighted twists tend to build up the muscle in your obliques, which, in turn, serves to thicken your waist. This diminishes your shoulder-to-waist differential, giving your physique a "blocky" appearance. Therefore, unless you have a naturally small waist, it is best to refrain from adding weights during exercise performance.

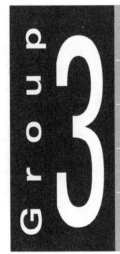

Group 3

ABDOMINAL exercises

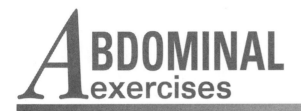
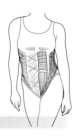

TRUNK TWIST

Begin by placing a bodybar behind your neck and allow it to rest across your shoulders. Wrap your arms around the bar and grasp each end to hold in position. Slowly twist your upper body to the right as far as possible, contracting your oblique muscles as you turn. Then, reverse direction and twist your body all the way to the left in the same fashion. Only your waist should move during this maneuver, and your hips should be stationary at all times. In order to reduce torque to your neck, look straight ahead and do not allow your head to turn during exercise performance.

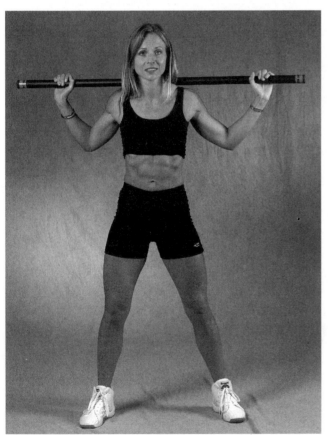

start

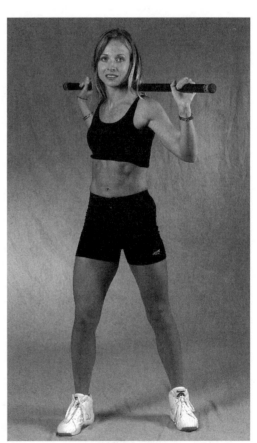

finish

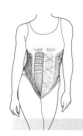

TWISTING CRUNCH

Begin by lying face up on the floor with your knees bent at a 90-degree angle. Your thighs should be perpendicular to the ground and your hands should be folded across your chest. Slowly raise your shoulders up and forward toward your chest, twisting your body to the right. Feel a contraction in the your abdominal muscles and then slowly reverse direction, returning to the start position. After performing the desired number of repetitions, repeat the process, twisting your body to the left.

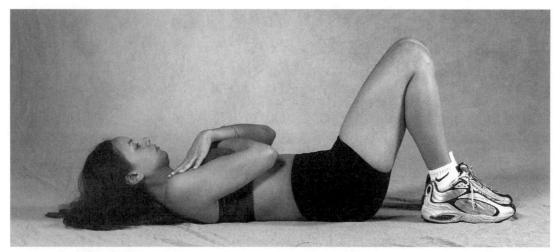

start

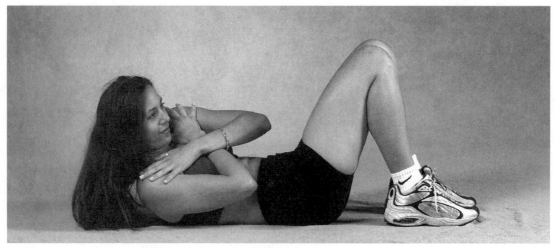

finish

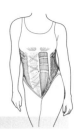

SWISS BALL SIDE BEND

Lie on your right side on top of a Swiss ball, placing your right hand at your right ear. Focus straight ahead and slowly bend your torso to the right as far as possible, bringing your right elbow toward your thigh. Make sure to bend only at the waist, leading with your shoulder and not your head. Contract your oblique muscles and then slowly return to the start position, keeping your body in alignment throughout the move. After performing the prescribed number of repetitions, repeat the process on the left.

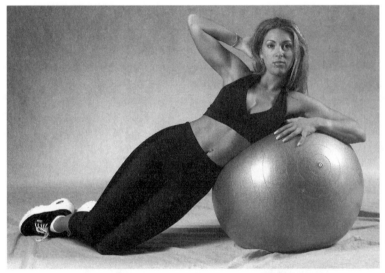

start

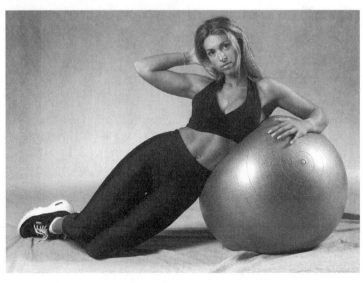

finish

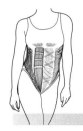

Abdominal exercises

REVERSE TRUNK TWIST

Begin by lying on your back with your arms out to the sides and palms on the floor. Keeping your legs straight and feet together, raise your thighs so that they are perpendicular with the ground. Slowly lower your legs directly to the right, keeping your torso pressed to the floor throughout the move. Raise your legs back to the start position and repeat the process on your left. Alternate from side to side for the desired number of repetitions.

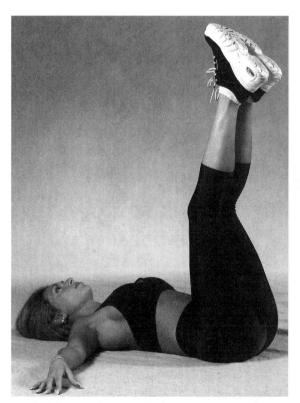

start

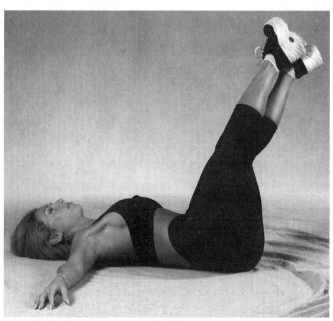

finish

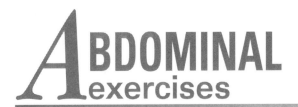

ABDOMINAL exercises

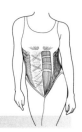

SIDE JACKKNIFE

Lie on your left side with your feet together. Make a fist with your right hand and keep it pressed to your ear. Simultaneously raise your right leg and torso toward each other as far as possible. Contract your oblique muscles and then slowly reverse direction and return to the start position. After performing the prescribed number of repetitions, repeat the process on the left.

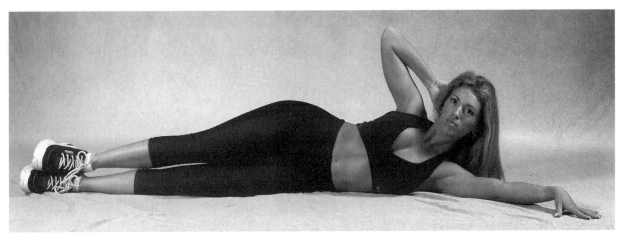

start

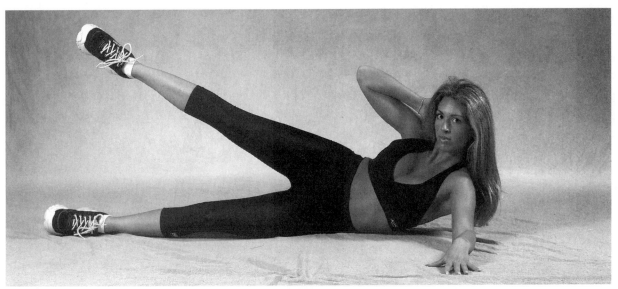

finish

Table 5.1 summarizes the abdominal exercises for each of the three groups.

TABLE 5.1

Group One	Group Two	Group Three
Crunch	Pelvic Tilt	Trunk Twist
Lying Machine Crunch	Reverse Curl	Twisting Crunch
Kneeling Rope Crunch	Hanging Knee Raise	Swiss Ball Side Bend
Seated Machine Curl	Pedaling	Reverse Trunk Twist
Toe Touch	Alternate Hanging Knee Raise	Side Jackknife

TIGHT BUNS

No part of the body attracts more attention than the glutes. Whether you're wearing tight-fitting jeans or a skimpy bikini, a well-shaped butt is sure to be an eye-catcher. It is the bodypart most identified with sex appeal and delineates the contours of your physique. And, of course, you can't look great naked without a great set of buns.

Sadly, the butt usually is the first area to lose its shape and definition. As you age, your glutes begin to atrophy (decrease in size), resulting in a corresponding loss of strength. When these muscles weaken, they gradually become unable to support the weight of your posterior. In the absence of exercise, your butt succumbs to the effects of gravity and begins a downward descent. The end result: a droopy, dumpy backside.

Frequently, women refuse to acknowledge that their glutes have gone south. They'll do everything possible to ignore this fate. When looking in the mirror, some even go so far as to avoid viewing themselves from behind. Self-denial, however, only serves to make things worse. Simply neglecting a problem area won't make it go away. Only by taking corrective action can you counteract the ravages of time and reverse the aging process.

Without question, attaining a toned tush is a difficult endeavor. The gluteal region is a storehouse for bodyfat, containing an abundance of adipose cells. From a functional standpoint, lower body fat serves a dual purpose. First, it acts as an energy reserve in anticipation of pregnancy and lactation. Second, it helps to cushion the posterior aspect of your pelvic bone (a bone called the ischium) so you can sit down in relative comfort. Because of these factors, the body tends to hold onto fat in this area. While it's one of the first places for fat to accumulate, it's generally the last to lose it (the first-in/last-out phenomenon).

To a certain extent, genetics will determine the size of your posterior. While some women are predisposed to a voluptuous physique with wide hips and lots of curves, others have more of an athletic build that's characterized by a fairly even distribution of body weight. These inherited attributes are immutable; for better or for worse, you can't change your basic physical structure. However, by target training the glutes within your individual framework, there is virtually no limit as to what *can* be accomplished. If your butt is flat, you can add shape and give it a rounded appearance. If your cheeks hang low, you can build them up to provide a natural lift. And if you have a little too much jiggle in your wiggle, you can enhance muscle tone to achieve a rock-hard look. Regardless of your present condition, a firm, shapely backside can be yours—provided you're willing to put in the effort.

In order to get your rear in gear, it is essential to isolate your glutes during training. Only by establishing a keen mind-to-muscle connection with these muscles will you realize the fruits of your labor. Because they are obscured from immediate view, most women are unable to contract their glutes effectively. In fact, many don't even perceive that their derriere is actually made up of muscle! They'll perform set after set of donkey kicks or pelvic lifts without really stimulating the area. Unfortunately, those who train in this fashion are doomed to failure. When performing any glute exercises, you must actively squeeze your butt on each rep, forcing it to contract. With consistent practice, you'll notice a big difference in the quality of your workouts and literally leave your glute troubles behind.

The exercises that follow are designed to target your glutes and hamstrings in combination. The glutes and hams maintain a symbiotic relationship. They both have attachments at the pelvic bone and interact to perform a variety of movements involving the hip joint. Consequently, it is beneficial to train these two muscles as a single entity, working them in concert with one another.

Anatomy of the Butt and Hamstrings

The butt and hamstrings comprise many individual muscles. Let's take a look at the form and function of the major muscles in this region:

➠ The gluteal group consists of three separate muscles: the **gluteus maximus, gluteus medius,** and **gluteus minimus**. The gluteus maximus is the largest of the gleateal muscles, accounting for the majority of muscular mass in the buttocks. Hence, the overall shape of your butt is largely determined by the development of this muscle. Its primary function is to extend the hip joint, allowing you to straighten your torso and bring your leg backward. The gluteus medius and gluteus minimus reside underneath and to the sides of the gluteus maximus. Their primary function is to bring the legs out and to the sides (a movement called abduction). Collectively, these muscles accentuate gluteal definition as well as firm up the hips.

➠ The hamstring complex consists of three separate muscles: the **biceps femoris, semitendinosis,** and **semimembranosus**. All three muscles essentially operate in concert with one another, helping both to extend the torso and flex the knee. They reside on the posterior aspect of the legs, originating at the hip and extending all the way down below the knee. Because these muscles are often very tight, they are particularly susceptible to pulls and strains. Thus, extra attention to flexibility training is needed to prevent an injury to this area.

Butt and Hamstrings "Dos and Don'ts"

The following are common mistakes made during glute training that should be explicitly avoided.

➠ ***Don't*** *overextend your hip joint:* In an effort to contract the glutes fully, women tend to overextend their hip joints (bring them too far behind the body). However, only a limited amount of hyperextension is possible at the hip. Past a certain point, stress is taken away from the target muscles of the glutes and is transferred to the lower back. Not only is this counterproductive to achieving glute definition, but it places undue stress on the hip joint and lumbar region, potentially leading to serious injury.

➠ ***Do*** concentrate on keeping constant tension on your glutes. Once you feel an intense contraction, reverse direction and begin the next rep.

➠ ***Don't*** *twist your body to complete a rep:* It is human nature to complete a task with the least amount of effort possible. Subconsciously, the body tries to gain leverage during training by using ancillary muscles for assistance. In many glute exercises, this is accomplished by contorting the upper body. When your torso is twisted, excessive torsion forces are placed on the vertebral column, often leading to disc rupture.

➠ ***Do*** maintain strict form, moving only the required muscles. To get the most out of your efforts, it is essential to resist the temptation to use leverage.

Figure 6.1provides an anatomical diagram that delineates the location of the gluteal and hamstrings muscles.

FIGURE 6.1

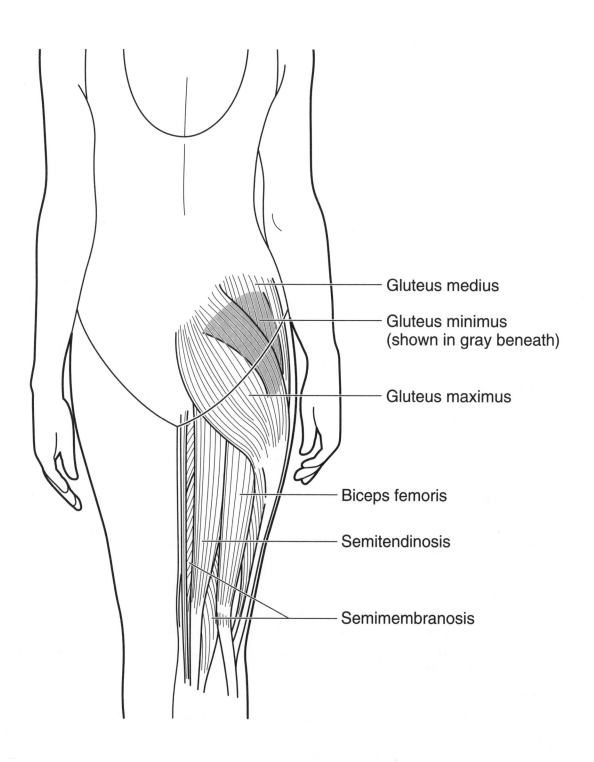

Buns exercises

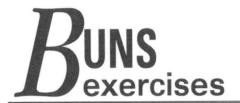
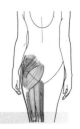

Group One

Group One exercises work your glutes and hamstrings in conjunction with one another. This is accomplished by performing movements that straighten your body from a bent position (extending your hips). These exercises are excellent for adding shape to your posterior, as well as for developing glute/ham stabilizer muscles that are a true sign of superior physical development.

Group One exercises, however, are limited by the strength of your lower back muscles (spinal erectors). Since the spinal erectors contribute to straightening your body from a bent position, they are highly involved in the performance of these movements. To minimize the stress to your lower back, it is imperative that you retain a lordotic curve (slight hyperextension of the lower back), keeping your lumbar area tight throughout each move. Not only will this develop the erectors, but it also alleviates pressure on the lumbar spine, helping to protect it from serious injury.

If you have incurred a previous injury to the lower back, it is recommended that you initially perform only nonweighted movements. In this way, you will safely stimulate the hamstrings and glutes while simultaneously strengthening the muscles of the lower back. Only after you have developed sufficient strength in your erectors should weighted movements be integrated into your routine.

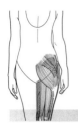
STIFF-LEGGED DEADLIFT

Stand with your feet shoulder width apart. Grasp two dumbbells and let them hang in front of your body. Keeping your knees straight, slowly bend forward at the hips and lower the dumbbells until you feel an intense stretch in your hamstrings. Then, reverse direction, contracting your glutes as you rise upward to the starting position.

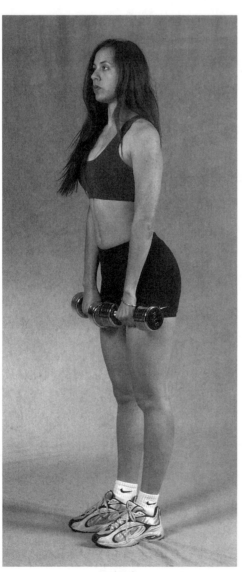

start

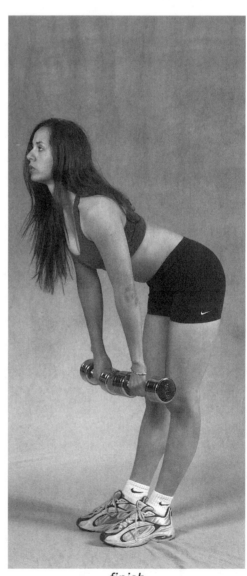

finish

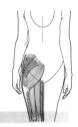

GOOD MORNING

Begin by resting a barbell across your shoulders. Assume a shoulder-width stance and keep your lower back taut throughout the movement. Slowly bend forward at the hips until your body is roughly parallel with the floor. In a controlled fashion, slowly reverse direction, contracting your glutes as you raise your body up along the same path back to the start position.

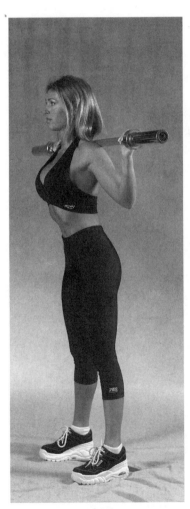

start

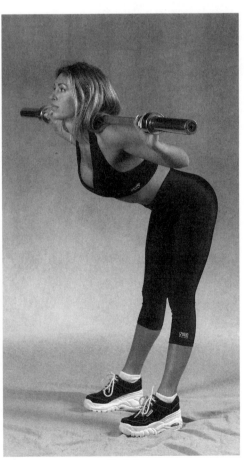

finish

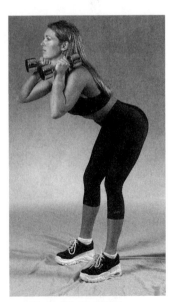

▲ *For Home Use:*
Grasp two dumbbells and hold them on your shoulders. Perform move as described.

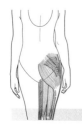

GLUTE/HAM RAISE

Begin by lying prone in a glute/ham machine with your thighs resting on the restraint pad and your heels hooked under the rollers. Keep your hands across your chest and arch your lower back. Slowly raise your torso upward until it is just short of parallel with the floor. Contract your glutes and then reverse direction, returning to the start position.

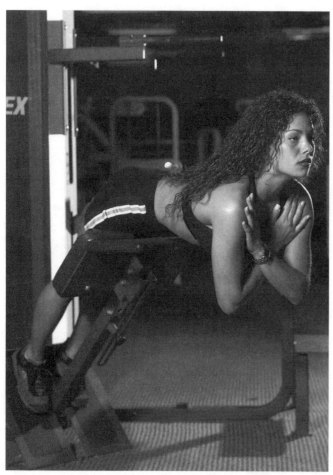

start

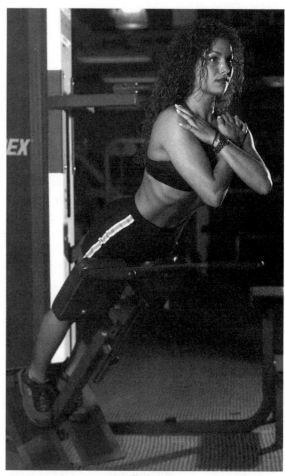

finish

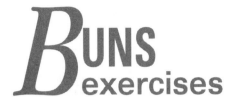 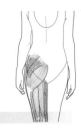

BUNS exercises

REVERSE HYPEREXTENSION

Begin by lying face down on a flat bench with your lower torso hanging off the end of the bench and your feet just short of touching the floor. Grasp the sides of the bench with both hands to support your body. Slowly raise your feet upward until they are just short of parallel with the ground, contracting your glutes at the top of the move. Then, reverse direction and return your legs to the start position.

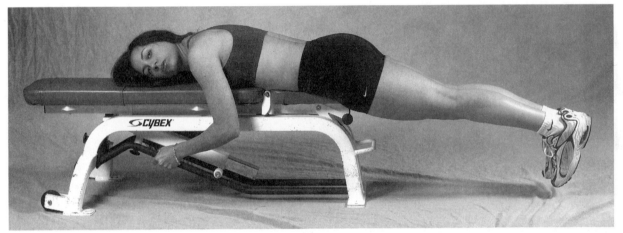

start

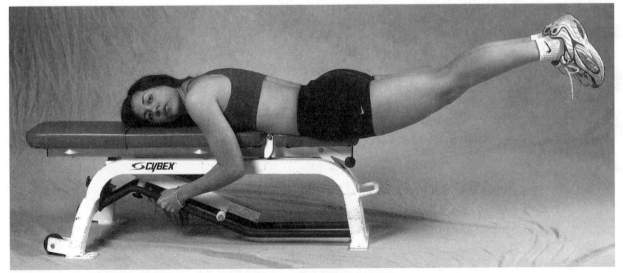

finish

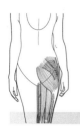

UNILATERAL HIP EXTENSION

Begin by placing your left knee on the bottom of an incline bench. Bend your elbows and place your forearms across the top of the bench so they support your body weight. Slowly raise your right leg as high as comfortably possible, keeping it straight throughout the move. Contract your glutes and then reverse direction, returning back to the start position. After performing the desired number of repetitions, repeat the process on your left.

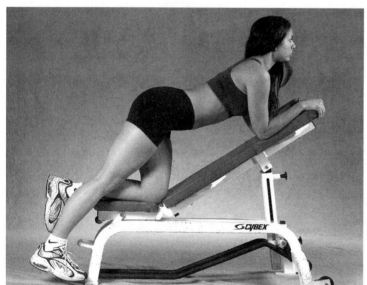

start

finish

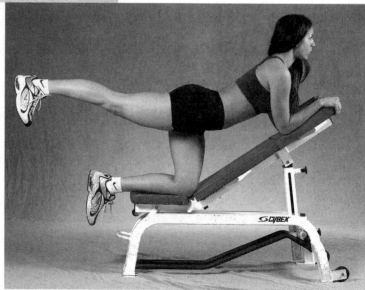

BUNS exercises

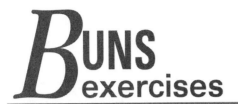
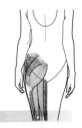

Group Two

Group Two exercises focus on the hamstrings, with minimal activation of the glutes. This is accomplished by performing knee flexion movements (i.e., bringing your heel up and back toward your butt). These exercises really help to firm up the back of the thigh—an area that is prone to jiggle.

In order to maximize hamstring activity, it is beneficial to point your feet downward throughout the course of each move, as if you were rising up on your toes (a movement called plantar flexion). This will reduce the involvement of your calf muscles during exercise performance (the calf muscles only can assist in knee flexion when they are stretched) and thereby allow the hamstrings to assume most of the work.

Additionally, by altering your leg position, you can shift emphasis to either the outer or the inner portion of your hamstrings. If you want to accentuate the outer hamstrings (biceps femoris), turn your legs out as you flex your knee (this is called lateral rotation). Alternatively, if you want to place more stress on the inner hamstrings, rotate your legs in during the movement (this is called medial rotation). Finally, keeping your legs straight will provide equal stimulation to all the hamstring muscles.

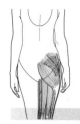

LYING LEG CURL

Begin by lying face down on a lying leg curl machine, with your heels hooked underneath the roller pads. Keeping your thighs pressed to the machine's surface, slowly curl your feet upward, stopping just short of touching your butt or as far as comfortably possible. Contract your hamstrings and then reverse direction, returning back to the start position.

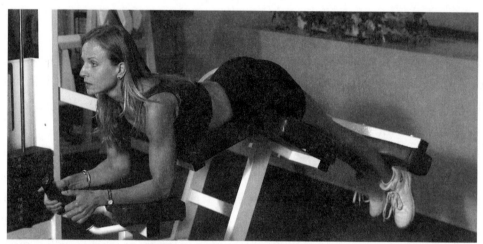

start

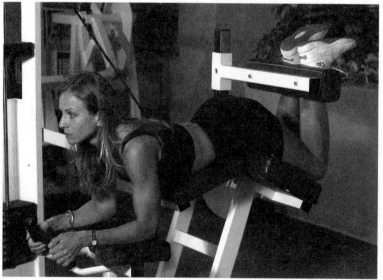

finish

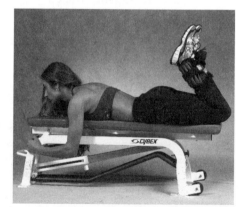

▲ ***For Home Use:*** Attach ankle weights to both ankles. Lie down on a bench and perform the move as described.

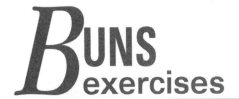 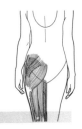

BUNS exercises

SEATED LEG CURL

Begin by sitting in a seated leg curl machine and place your heels over the roller pads. Lower the leg restraint over your thighs so that they are secure. Slowly press your feet downward as far as comfortably possible, contracting your hamstrings when your knees are fully bent. Then, reverse direction and return to the start position.

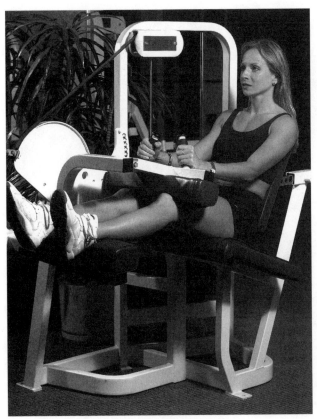

start

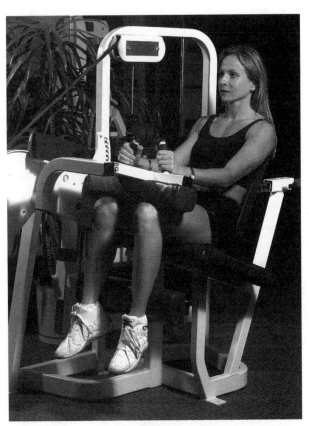

finish

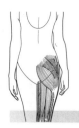

STANDING LEG CURL

Begin by attaching an ankle weight to your right ankle. Grasp onto a stationary object and slowly curl your right foot upward, stopping just short of touching your butt or as far as comfortably possible. Contract your right hamstring and then reverse direction, returning back to the start position. After performing the desired number of repetitions, repeat the process on your left.

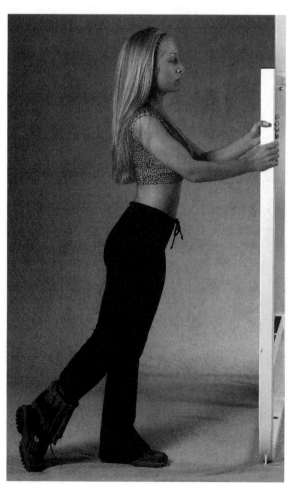

start

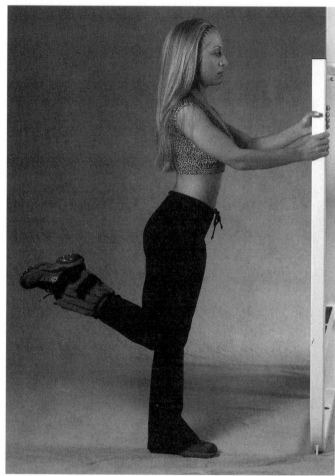

finish

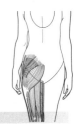

Kneeling leg curl

Begin by kneeling in a kneeling leg curl machine, placing your right heel underneath the roller pad. Place your forearms on the restraint pads for support. Slowly curl your right foot upward, stopping just short of touching your butt or as far as comfortably possible. Contract your right hamstring and then reverse direction, returning to the start position. After performing the desired number of repetitions, repeat the process on your left.

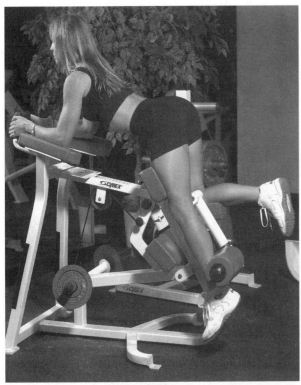

start

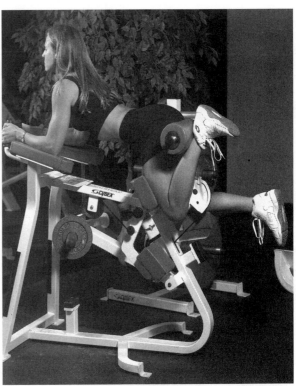

finish

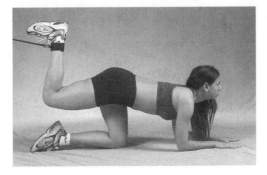

For Home Use: Attach a strength band to a stationary object and then fasten it to your right ankle. Kneel on the floor with your right leg extended and perform the move as described.

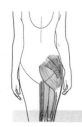

Buns exercises

CABLE LEG CURL

Begin by attaching a cuff to a low cable pulley and then securing the cuff to your right ankle. Position yourself so that you are facing the weight stack and grasp a sturdy portion of the machine for support. Slowly curl your right foot upward, stopping just short of touching your butt or as far as comfortably possible. Contract your right hamstring and then reverse direction, returning to the start position. After performing the desired number of repetitions, repeat the process on your left.

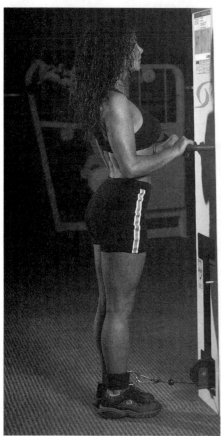

start   *finish*

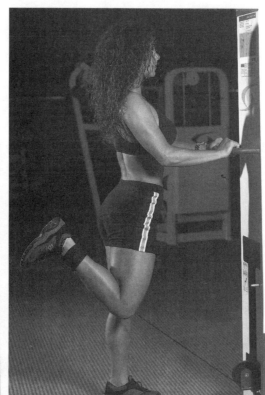

For Home Use: Attach a strength band to a stationary object and then fasten it to your right ankle. Grab on to the stationary object and perform the move as described. ▶

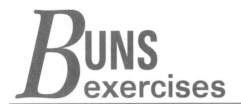

Buns exercises

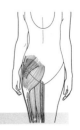

Group Three

Group Three exercises focus on the glutes, with only minimal activation of the hamstrings. This is accomplished by performing abduction movements (i.e., bringing your leg away from the midline of your body). Specifically, these exercises target the gluteus medius and gluteus minimus, which are often overpowered by the much larger gluteus maximus. Hence, superior gluteal shape is achieved.

You can achieve additional posterior development by turning your legs out (lateral rotation) during abduction. This activates a group of muscles called the external rotators (including the piriformis, quadratus femoris, and several other muscles). Although small in size, these muscles are important both from a functional, as well as an aesthetic, perspective.

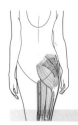

CABLE ABDUCTOR PULL

Begin by attaching a cuff to a low cable pulley and then securing the cuff to your right ankle. Position yourself so that your left side faces the weight stack and grasp a sturdy portion of the machine for support. Pull your right leg across your body and directly out to the side. Contract your glutes and then slowly return the weight along the same path back to the start position. After finishing the desired number of repetitions, invert the process and repeat on the left.

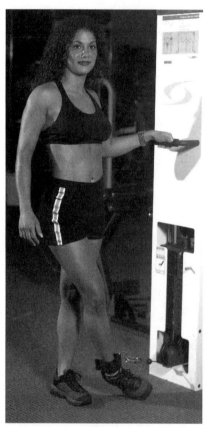

start

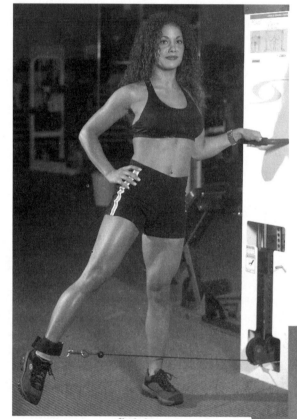

finish

For Home Use: Attach a strength band to a stationary object and then fasten it to your ankle. Grasp the stationary object and perform the move as described. ▶

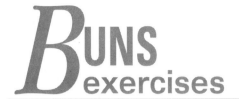

BUNS exercises

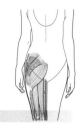

SEATED MACHINE ABDUCTION

Begin by sitting in an abductor machine and, with your legs together, place your outer thighs on the restraint pads. Slowly force your legs apart as far as comfortably possible. Contract your glutes and then reverse direction, returning to the start position.

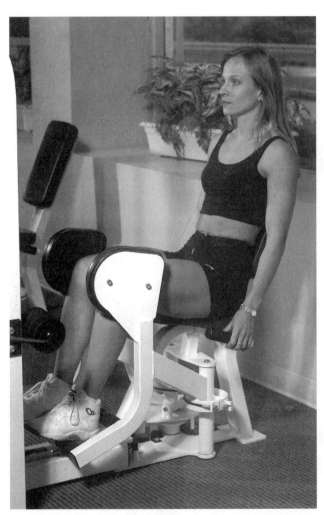

start

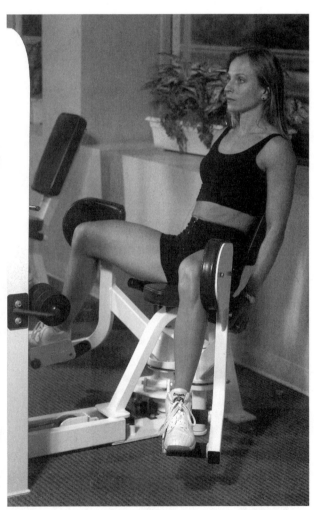

finish

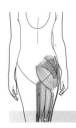

BUNS exercises

STANDING ABDUCTION

Begin by attaching an ankle weight to your right ankle. Stand with your feet together and grasp a sturdy, stationary object for support. Bring your right leg directly out to the side as far as comfortably possible. Contract your glutes and then slowly return the weight along the same path back to the start position. After finishing the desired number of repetitions, invert the process and repeat on the left.

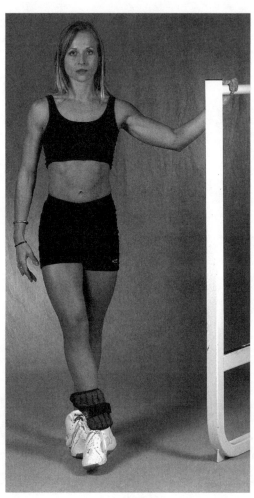

start

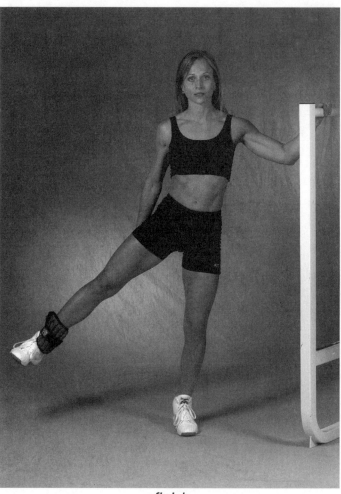

finish

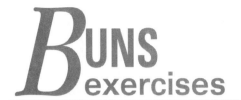 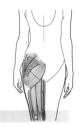

BUNS exercises

LYING ABDUCTION

Begin by lying down on your left side. Bend your left leg at a 90-degree angle and bring your left foot to rest underneath your right knee. Keeping your right leg straight, slowly raise it as high as possible. Contract your glutes and return to the start position. After finishing the desired number of repetitions, turn over and repeat the process on your left.

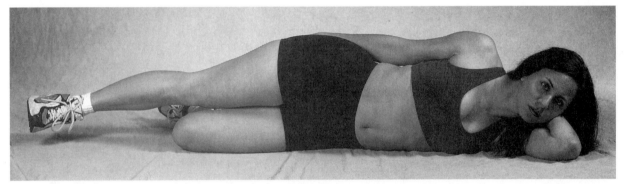

start

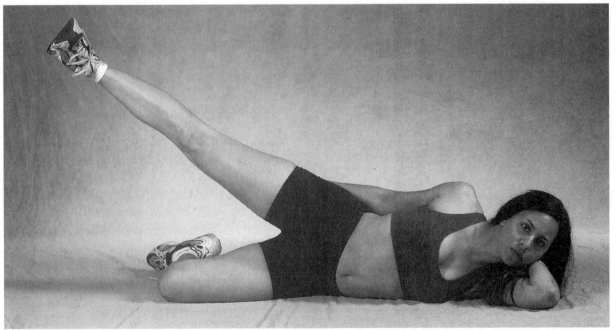

finish

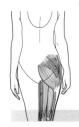

KNEELING ABDUCTION

Begin by kneeling on the ground, assuming an "all-fours" position. Keeping your right leg bent, raise it to the side as high as comfortably possible. Contract your glutes and then slowly return the weight along the same path back to the start position. After finishing the desired number of repetitions, repeat the process on your left.

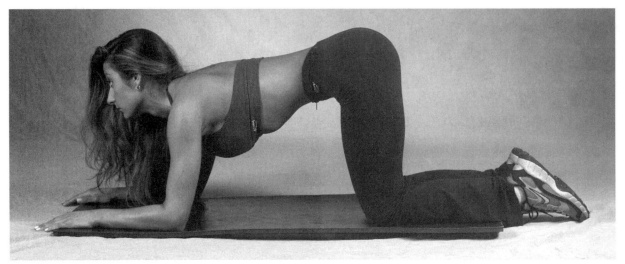

start

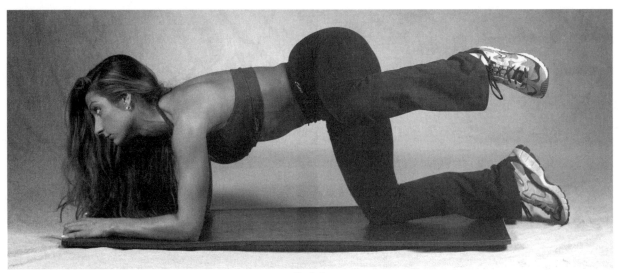

finish

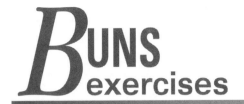 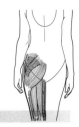

Table 6.1 summarizes the glute and hamstrings exercises for each of the three groups.

TABLE 6.1

Group One	Group Two	Group Three
Stiff-Legged Deadlift	Lying Leg Curl	Cable Abductor Pull
Good Morning	Seated Leg Curl	Seated Machine Abduction
Glute/Ham Raise	Standing Leg Curl	Standing Abduction
Reverse Hyperextension	Kneel Leg Curl	Lying Abduction
Unilateral Hip Extension	Cable Leg Curl	Kneeling Abduction

SHAPELY THIGHS

A woman's thighs can be her greatest physical asset— or her biggest bane. Throughout the ages, the thighs have epitomized the female physique. Although standards may have changed over time, they have always been a symbol of female beauty and a source of male desire.

Poorly developed thighs inevitably lead to "thigh anxiety"—a fear of exposing your legs in public. When your thighs are out of shape, your options for dress are limited. The only way to hide them is by wearing loose, baggy pants or sweats—not exactly the most flattering of attire. You certainly can't put on anything tight. Short skirts are out. A bathing suit? No way. Inevitably, your wardrobe is confined to nothing but demure, matronly apparel.

On the other hand, a great set of thighs makes shopping for clothes a breeze. They are the most visible of all the trouble zones and can be displayed in a myriad of ways. Whether you wear the miniest of miniskirts, the shortest of shorts, or any other revealing bottom, sexy thighs are a bare necessity. And the less you have on, the better they look!

In certain cases, only specific parts of the thighs are problematic. Some women have trouble with their inner thighs, others with their upper thighs, and still others with the region around their knees. If this is your predicament, don't fret: Targeted bodysculpting can isolate these areas and tone them to perfection.

Attaining excellent thigh shape is generally not a difficult proposition. By nature, women tend to have muscular legs. In fact, while men are much stronger than women in the upper body, innate lower body strength is fairly equal between the sexes. This phenomenon is necessary for childbirth. Women must have sufficient capacity to carry a fetus throughout term. Consequently, the legs usually respond well to exercise. Once bodyfat has been stripped away, the thighs can be shaped more easily than virtually any other bodypart.

However, although results can be achieved readily, expect to put a lot of hard work into your routine. Thigh training is a grueling experience that necessitates a great deal of intestinal fortitude. Since the thighs are the largest muscle complex in the body, they require a substantial amount of energy to sustain exercise performance. After an intense set, your heart will be pounding and you'll be gasping for air. No other muscle group is quite so physically demanding. Fortunately, these aftereffects subside within a short period of time. And, once your workout is finished, you can take solace in the fact that you'll soon have thighs to die for.

Anatomy of the Thighs

The frontal thighs comprise many individual muscles. Let's take a look at the form and function of the major muscles in this region:

➡ The quadriceps consists of four separate muscles: the **rectus femoris, vastus lateralis, vastus medialis,** and **vastus intermedius**. All four of these muscles have an attachment at the quadriceps tendon on the knee. The three vastus muscles originate on the femur (thighbone). The rectus femoris, on the other hand, originates at the hip, making it a two-joint muscle—a fact that enhances its bodysculpting capabilities.

➡ The adductors consist of three separate muscles: the **adductor brevis, adductor longus,** and **adductor magnus**. These are the primary muscles of the inner thigh. Not only are the adductors important from an aesthetic standpoint, but they help to stabilize the lower body and promote an erect posture.

Figure 7.1 provides an anatomic diagram that delineates the location of the muscles of the hips and thighs.

FIGURE 7.1

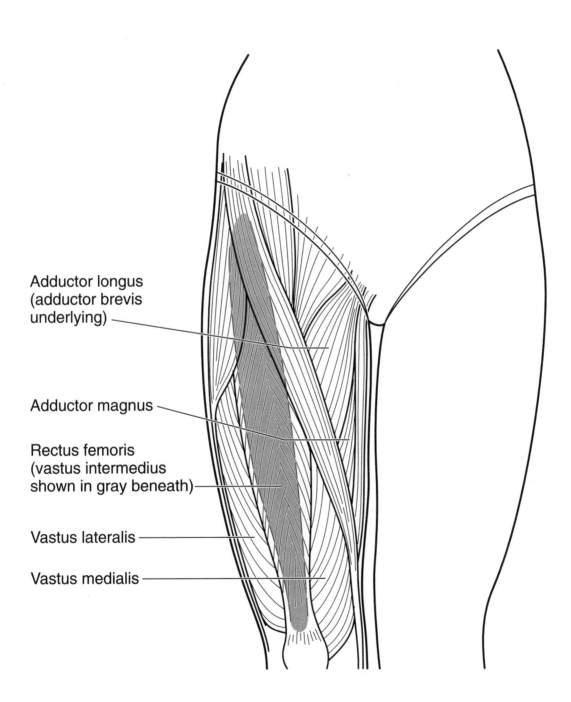

Adductor longus (adductor brevis underlying)

Adductor magnus

Rectus femoris (vastus intermedius shown in gray beneath)

Vastus lateralis

Vastus medialis

Thigh "Dos and Don'ts"

The following are common mistakes made during thigh training that should be explicitly avoided.

➠ ***Don't*** *lock out your knees when training your thighs:* All too frequently, women completely straighten their legs at the finish of a rep. However, not only does this take stimulation away from the thigh muscles, it also places a great deal of stress directly on the joints.

➠ ***Do*** stop just short of lockout, keeping continuous tension on your thighs at all times. There always should be a slight bend in your knees at the finish position of each move.

➠ ***Don't*** *overexaggerate foot position when training your thighs:* In an effort to work various aspects of the frontal thigh, it is common to turn the feet in or out during exercise performance. However, the benefits of this practice are rather subtle, and the overall effect will be limited. Certainly, you should avoid exaggerating these foot positions, as it can cause damage to the knee. This is especially important during closed chain movements where the feet are immobile (such as the squat, leg press, etc.).

➠ ***Do*** keep your feet turned slightly outward during all closed-chain movements (such as the squat and leg press). Doing so allows the patella (knee) to move in its natural arc, maintaining the integrity of the joint. If you choose to experiment with different foot positions, do so only in open chain movements, (such as the leg extension) and make sure to stay in a comfortable range.

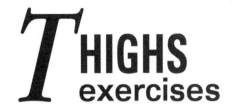

THIGHS
exercises

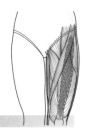

Group One

Group One exercises focus on overall thigh development. This is accomplished by performing basic, compound movements that employ both hip and knee extension (i.e., straightening the knees and hips from a bent position). The quads and adductors are all heavily involved in these exercises. In addition, many of the stabilizer muscles in the lower body (and even some in the upper body) also are activated.

Without question, Group One exercises are both physically and mentally challenging. Because of their multijoint nature, skill and coordination are needed for proper execution. Accordingly, these movements should be performed as the first exercise in your thigh workout, when your energy levels are at their peak.

It is important to avoid allowing your knees to travel over your toes during the performance of these maneuvers. Since the structure of the knees provides for only a limited range of forward movement, going past this point can readily cause damage to the joint's connective tissue.

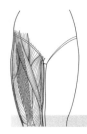

THIGHS exercises

SQUAT

Begin by resting a straight bar high on the back of your neck. Assume a shoulder-width stance, grasping the bar with both hands. Slowly lower your body until your thighs are parallel with the ground. Your lower back should be slightly arched and your heels should stay in contact with the floor at all times. When you reach a "seated" position, reverse direction by straightening your legs and return to the start position.

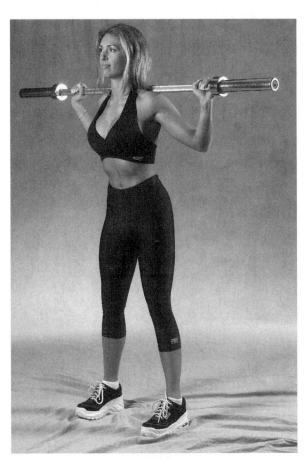

start

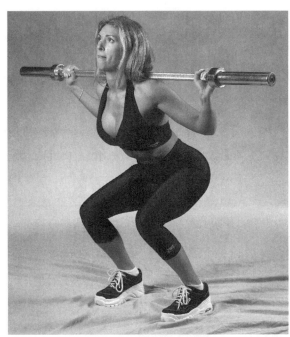

finish

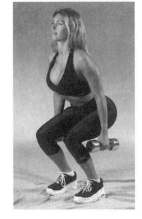

For Home Use: Grasp two dumbbells and allow them to rest gently at your sides. Perform the move as described. ▶

*T*HIGHS
exercises

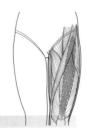

LEG PRESS

Begin by sitting in a leg press machine, keeping your back pressed firmly into the padded seat. Place your feet on the footplate with a shoulder-width stance. Straighten your legs and unlock the carriage release bars located on the sides of the machine. Slowly lower your legs, bringing your knees into your chest. Without bouncing at the bottom, press the weight up in a controlled fashion, stopping just short of locking out your knees. Contract your quads and then return the weight to the start position.

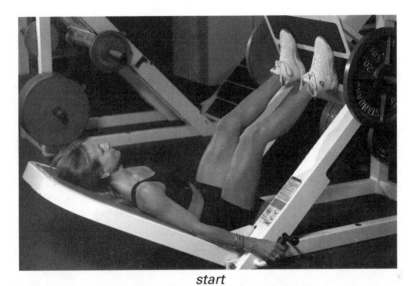

start

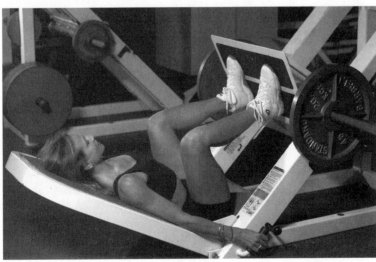

finish

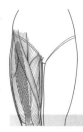

*T*HIGHS
exercises

STEP-UP

Begin by grasping a pair of dumbbells and allow them to hang at your sides. Stand facing the side of a flat bench with your feet shoulder width apart. Pushing off your right leg, step up with your left foot and follow with your right foot so that both feet are flat on the bench. Step back down in the same order, first with your left foot and then with your right, returning to the start position.

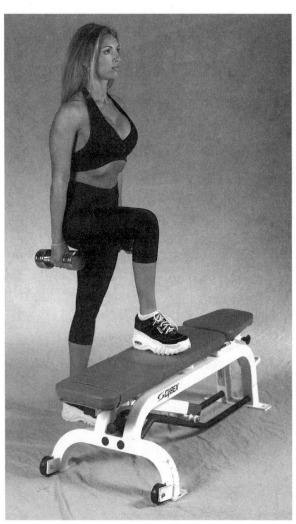

start

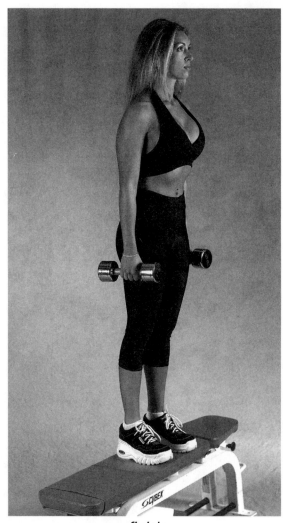

finish

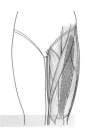

*T*HIGHS
exercises

FRONT SQUAT

Begin by resting a straight bar across your upper chest, holding it in place with both hands. Assuming a shoulder-width stance, slowly lower your body until your thighs are parallel with the ground. Your lower back should be slightly arched and your heels should stay in contact with the floor at all times. When you reach a "seated" position, reverse direction by straightening your legs and return to the start position.

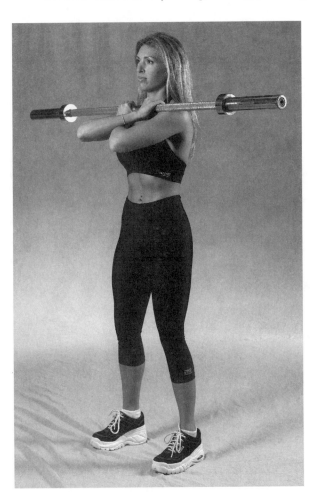

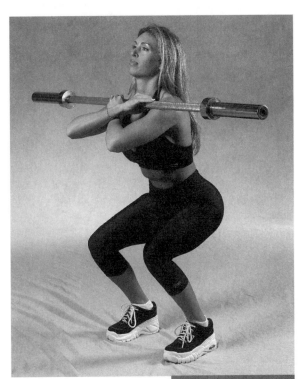

For Home Use: Grasp two dumbbells and, with your palms facing toward your body, hold them across your chest at shoulder level. Perform the move as described. ▶

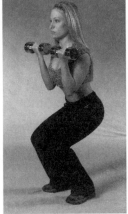

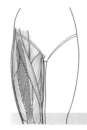

LUNGE

Begin by grasping two dumbbells and allow them to hang down by your sides. Take a long stride forward with your right leg and raise your left heel so that your left foot is on its toes. Keeping your shoulders back and chin up, slowly lower your body by flexing your right knee and hip, continuing your descent until your right knee is almost in contact with floor. Reverse direction by forcibly extending the right hip and knee until you return to the start position. After performing the desired number of reps, repeat the process on your left. For a greater effect, you can perform walking lunges, where you continue lunging forward until the desired number of reps is completed.

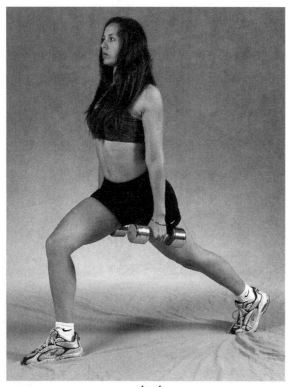

start

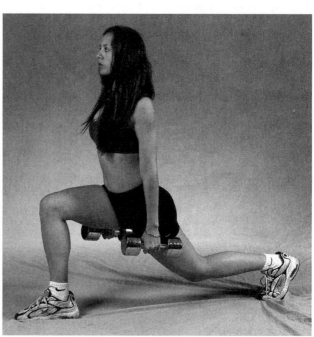

finish

*T*HIGHS
exercises

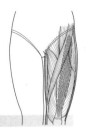

Group Two

Group Two exercises are isolation movements that target specific areas of the frontal thigh. This is accomplished by performing movements that either extend the knee or flex the hip. Because of their single-joint orientation, these exercises primarily work the quadriceps muscles without significant effect on the other thigh musculature.

The vastus muscles are most active in exercises that involve knee extension (straightening the knee from a bent position). It is common for women to have "knobby" knees, which impairs the natural sweep of the thighs. Developing the vastus muscles can help to define this area and accentuate your proportions.

Alternatively, the upper portion of the quadriceps (rectus femoris) is more active in movements that involve hip flexion (raising the leg upward, as in a kicking motion). Since the upper thigh is one of the more difficult areas to develop, significant attention must be given to improve this area in order to achieve optimal shape and definition.

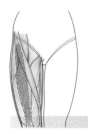

*T*HIGHS
exercises

LEG EXTENSIONS

Begin by sitting back in a leg extension machine. Bend your knees and place your instep underneath the roller pad located at the bottom of the machine. Grasp the machine's handles for support. Slowly bring your feet upward until your legs are just short of parallel with the ground. Contract your quads and then reverse direction, returning to the start position.

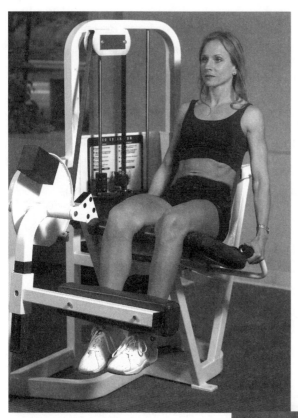

start

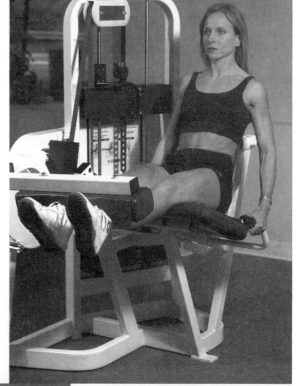

finish

For Home Use: Attach leg weights to your ankles and sit at the end of a flat bench. Perform the move as described. ▶

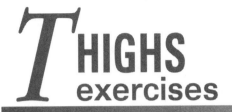
THIGHS exercises

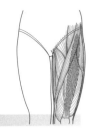

ONE-LEGGED LEG EXTENSIONS

Begin by sitting back in a leg extension machine. Bend your right knee and place your right instep underneath the roller pad located at the bottom of the machine. Grasp the machine's handles for support. Slowly bring your right foot upward until it is just short of parallel with the ground. Contract your right quad and then reverse direction, returning to the start position. After performing the desired number of reps, repeat the process on your left.

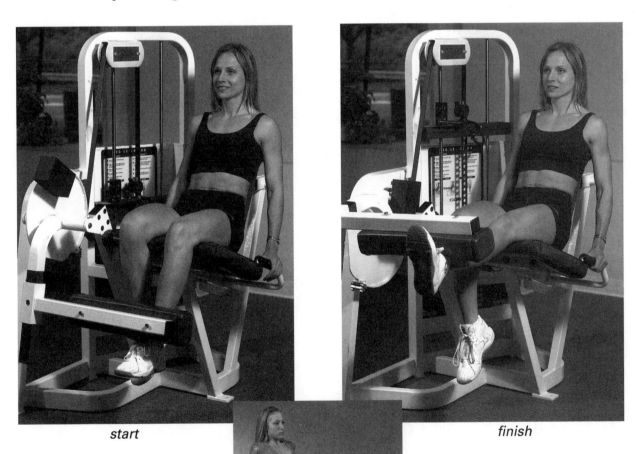

start

finish

For Home Use: Attach leg weights to your ankles and sit at the end of a flat bench. Perform the move as described. ▶

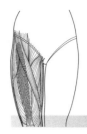

FRONT CABLE KICKS

Begin by attaching a cuff to a low cable pulley and then securing the cuff to your right ankle. Position yourself so that your body faces away from the apparatus and grasp a sturdy portion of the machine for support. Slowly bring your foot forward and up as high as possible, contracting your right quad at the top of the movement. Then, reverse direction and return your leg to the start position. After performing the desired number of reps, repeat the process on your left.

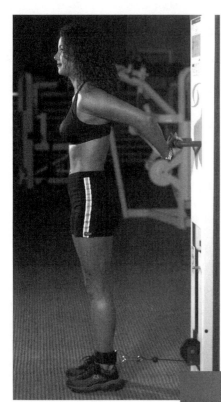

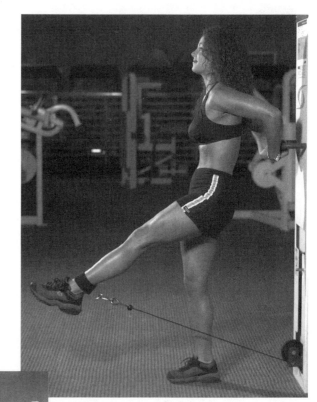

start

finish

◄ ***For Home Use:*** Attach one end of a strength band to a stationary object and attach the other end to your right ankle. Perform the move as described.

*T*HIGHS exercises

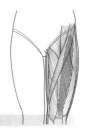

Sissy squat

Begin by taking a shoulder-width stance. Grasp an incline bench with one hand and rise onto your toes. In one motion, slowly slant your torso back, bend your knees and lower your body downward. Thrust your knees forward as you descend and lean back until your torso is almost parallel with the floor. Then, reverse direction and rise upward until you reach the starting position.

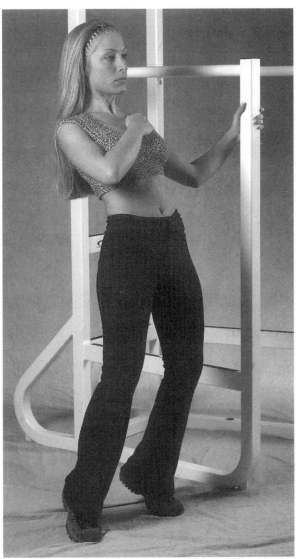

start

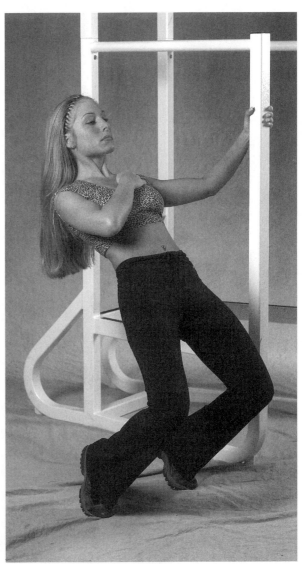

finish

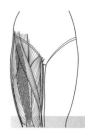

*T*HIGHS
exercises

SEATED SINGLE LEG LIFT

Begin by attaching a leg weight to your right ankle. Sit on the floor, leaning back slightly and supporting your weight with your hands. Bend your left knee and keep the left foot planted on the floor. Straighten your right leg and let it hang down a few inches from the ground. Slowly raise your right leg upward as far as comfortably possible. Contract your right quad and then reverse direction, returning to the start position. After performing the desired number of reps, repeat the process on your left.

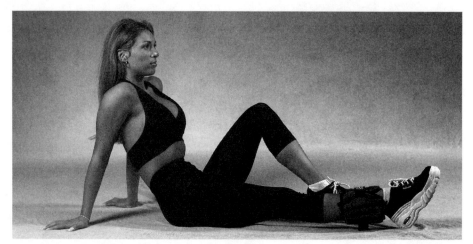

start

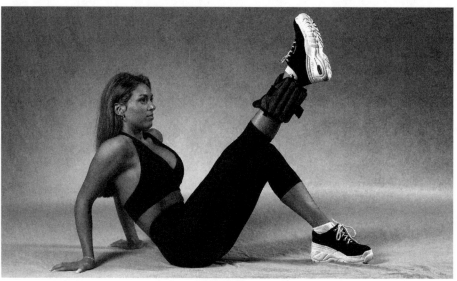

finish

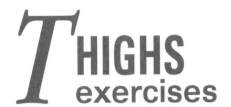 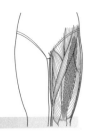

THIGHS exercises

Group Three

Group Three exercises target the inner thighs. This is accomplished by using adduction movements (bringing the thigh toward the midline of the body). As the name implies, these exercises work the adductors in relative isolation, helping to firm up the entire inner thigh region.

For most women, the inner thighs are especially problematic. Go into any gym and you'll see women lined up to use the adductor machines, believing this will solve their inner thigh dilemma. You must understand, however, that training your adductors won't strip away excess fat in the region. Remember, you cannot spot reduce! Only through a combination of proper nutrition and dedicated total-body exercise will the thigh fat disappear, revealing the lean, hard muscle that you've worked so hard to develop.

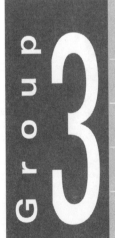

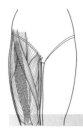

SEATED MACHINE ADDUCTION

Begin by sitting in an adductor machine and, with your legs spread apart, place your inner thighs on the restraint pads. Slowly force your legs together, contracting your inner thighs as the pads touch one another. Then, reverse direction and return to the start position.

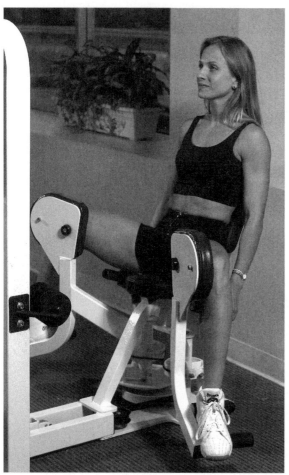

start

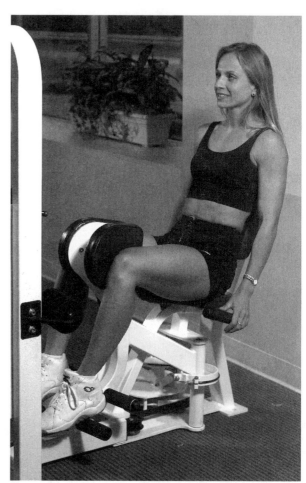

finish

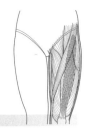

THIGHS exercises

ADDUCTOR CABLE PULLS

Begin by attaching a cuff to a low cable pulley and then securing the cuff to your right ankle. Position yourself so that your right side faces the weight stack and grasp a sturdy portion of the machine for support. Slowly pull your right leg toward and across the midline of your body, as far to the left as possible. Contract your inner thigh muscles and then reverse direction, returning your leg to the start position. After performing the desired number of reps, repeat the process on your left.

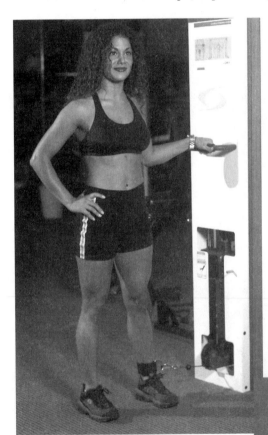

start

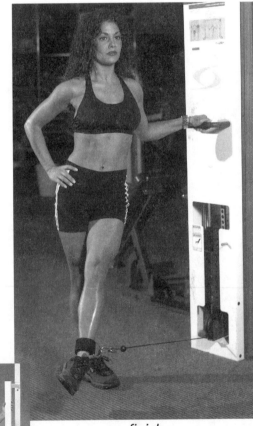

finish

For Home Use: Attach one end of a strength band to a stationary object and attach the other end to your right ankle. Perform the move as described. ▶

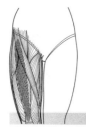

SIDE LUNGE

Begin by assuming a stance slightly wider than shoulder width. Grasp two dumbbells and hold one in front and one in back of your body. Keeping your left leg straight, slowly bend your right knee out to the side until your right thigh is parallel with the floor. Then, slowly rise back up and repeat this process immediately on your left.

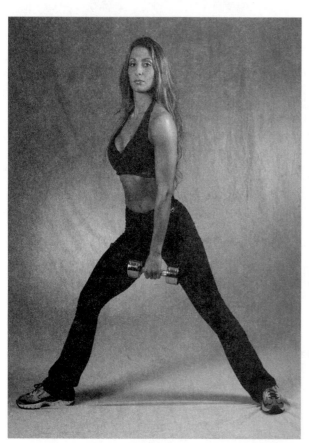

start

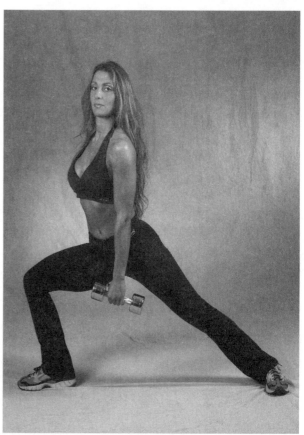

finish

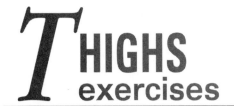

THIGHS
exercises

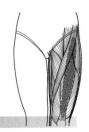

LYING ADDUCTOR RAISE

Begin by lying down on your right side. Bring your left leg over your right leg, keeping it bent at a 90 degree angle with your left foot planted firmly on the floor. Keeping your right leg straight, slowly raise it as high as possible. Contract your inner thigh and return to the start position. After finishing the desired number of repetitions, turn over and repeat the process on your left. For added intensity, attach ankle weights.

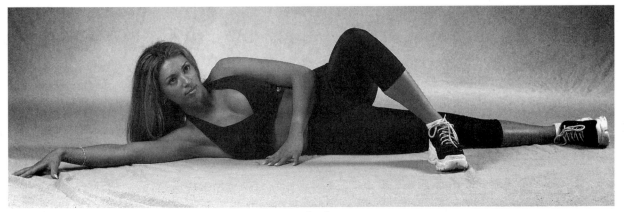

start

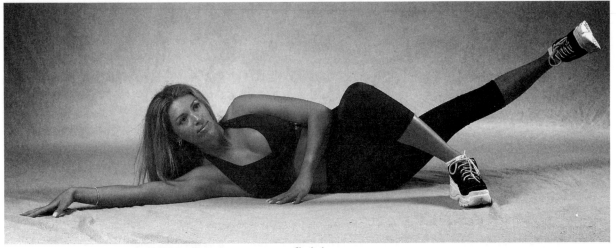

finish

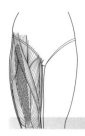

SEATED INSIDE RAISE

Begin by sitting on the floor, leaning back slightly and supporting your weight on your hands. Bend your left leg and keep your left foot planted firmly on the floor. Extend your right leg as far to the side as comfortably possible. Keeping your right leg straight, pull it up and in toward your left knee. Contract your inner thigh and then reverse direction, returning to the start position. After performing the desired number of reps, repeat the process on your left.

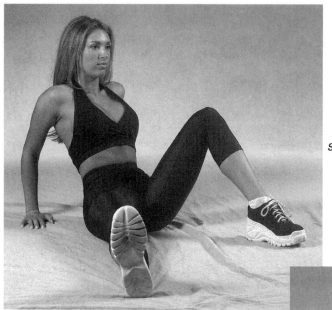

start

finish

Table 7.1 summarizes the thigh exercises for each of the three groups.

TABLE 7.1

Group One	Group Two	Group Three
Squat	Leg Extensions	Seated Machine Adduction
Leg Press	One-Legged Leg Extensions	Adductor Cable Pulls
Step Up	Front Cable Kicks	Side Lunge
Front Squat	Sissy Squat	Lying Adductor Raise
Lunge	Seated Single Leg Lift	Seated Inside Raise

STOKING THE FAT-BURNING FURNACE

If you're like the great majority of women, you've probably done some type of aerobic training at some point in your life. There's a good chance you've even performed aerobics on a regular basis. Whether it's jogging, biking, kickboxing, or any of the other dozens of cardiovascular activities, women gravitate to aerobics like bees to honey.

Unfortunately, aerobics are often misunderstood. There is a prevailing misconception that aerobics are the key to physical perfection: Just get on the treadmill or take a few classes and you'll turn your body into a work of art. However, aerobics actually do little to improve your muscular shape and hardness. Without targeted bodysculpting, you'll never develop appreciable muscle tone and your body will end up loose and flabby—even if it's devoid of bodyfat.

Nevertheless, aerobics are an important component in a fitness regimen. Besides having a positive impact on your cardiovascular health, aerobics also play a significant role in body aesthetics. Let's take a look at these benefits:

➠ *Aerobics expedite fat burning.* A large portion of the calories that are expended during aerobic training are derived from fat. Depending on your exercise intensity, a single session of cardio can burn more than 20 grams of fat—enough to offset the amount in a greasy burger and fries. But the fat-burning effects extend beyond the immediate. Your metabolism remains elevated even after you have finished training, prolonging fat burning for up to several hours after your session. Moreover, your mitochondria (cellular furnaces where fat burning takes place) expand in size and number, and your aerobic enzymes (chemical messengers that accelerate the fat-burning process) increase in quantity. Over time, these factors allow your body to rely more on utilizing fat, rather than glycogen (carbohydrates), for fuel, helping to sustain long-term weight management.

➠ *Aerobics improve muscular endurance.* When you lift weights, your body converts glucose into the high-energy compound adenosine triphosphate (through a process called glycolysis) to fuel exercise performance. During this conversion process, lactic acid is produced and rapidly accumulates in your muscles as you train. When lactic acid builds up past a certain point, you experience an intense burning sensation in your muscles. Ultimately, the burn becomes so strong that it inhibits your ability to continue training. However, by increasing aerobic capacity, your cardiovascular system becomes more efficient at delivering oxygen to your working muscles. This helps to increase your lactate threshold—the point at which there is more lactic acid in your body than can be metabolized—and thereby delays the onset of lactic acid buildup. The end result is a greater capacity to train at a high level of intensity.

➠ *Aerobics enhance muscular recuperation.* Aerobics help to expand your network of capillaries—the tiny blood vessels that allow nutrients such as protein and carbohydrates to be absorbed into body tissues. The more capillaries that you have, the more efficient your body becomes in utilizing these nutrients for muscular repair. Capillaries also help to clear waste products, particularly carbon dioxide, from the food burning process, further enhancing the efficiency of your nutrient delivery system. This accelerates the rate at which your muscles are able to get the resources needed for recuperation, helping to improve workouts and speed recovery.

Given these benefits, it would be remiss to exclude aerobics from your workout regimen. Aerobics provide the perfect complement to a strength training routine, helping you attain a lean, hard appearance. But to get the most out of aerobics, you need to adhere to certain guidelines. There is a science to aerobics, and only by following established protocols will you optimize results.

Frequency

Because cardiovascular exercise is endurance oriented, many women believe it can be performed on a daily basis. However, while it's true that your body can tolerate a greater volume of aerobic exercise (as opposed to anaerobic activity), too much of it eventually will set back your progress and have a negative impact on your physique. Only by striking the right balance between exercise and rest will you reap maximal rewards.

During the recovery period, your body is able to regenerate its glycogen reserves. Glycogen is your body's primary energy source, giving you the strength and endurance to perform physical activities. Since cardio burns glycogen (as well as fat) during exercise performance, these reserves eventually become depleted, leaving you tired and fatigued. Ultimately, your training ability is hampered, diminishing the quality of your workouts.

In extreme cases, performing an excess of aerobics can result in a condition called overtraining syndrome (OTS). Overtraining makes your body less efficient in utilizing fat for fuel and is apt to cannibalize your muscle tissue (due to a secretion of stress hormones) for energy. Moreover, it can throw off your biochemical balance, causing a variety of complications that include cessation of your period (amenorrhea), chronic fatigue, and other anomalies. To avoid this fate, you must constantly monitor your physical state, paying keen attention to the symptoms relating to overtraining (see the accompanying box). There is a fine line between training and overtraining; make sure you don't cross over it.

SYMPTOMS OF OVERTRAINING

Overtraining syndrome (OTS) is a common exercise-related affliction. Studies show that it affects as much as 10 percent of all people who exercise on a regular basis. Due to a lack of understanding about the subject, OTS often ends up going undiagnosed.

The following are some of the symptoms relating to overtraining. If you experience two or more of these symptoms, you might be overtrained. If symptoms persist, get plenty of sleep and don't resume training until you feel mentally and physically ready.

- ▶ *Increased resting heart rate*
- ▶ *Increased resting blood pressure*
- ▶ *Decreased exercise performance*
- ▶ *Decreased appetite*
- ▶ *Decreased desire to work out*
- ▶ *Increased incidence of injuries*
- ▶ *Increased incidence of infections and flulike symptoms*
- ▶ *Increased irritability and depression*

Depending on your individual situation, cardio should be performed between three and five days a week. You should assess your need to lose bodyfat and adjust the frequency of your aerobic training accordingly. Just make sure you don't overdo it. Allow your body at least two full days a week of complete rest from exercise. This will help to enhance recovery and ensure adequate regeneration of your energy supplies. When in doubt, err on the side of caution. Remember, with respect to exercise, less can be more!

Duration

You don't need to perform lengthy aerobic sessions to reduce bodyfat. I have seen women stay on the treadmill for hours on end. They are so consumed with losing weight that cardiovascular exercise assumes a significant portion of their day. However, not only is this unnecessary, it actually can be counterproductive. As long as you train properly, optimal results are achieved in a modicum of time.

During the initial stages of training, you may only be able to endure a few minutes of cardio. If you aren't aerobically conditioned, oxygen will be in short supply and you'll get winded rather easily. Don't let this get you down. Endurance tends to build up very rapidly. Within a few weeks, you'll see major improvements in your stamina and, before long, cardio will be a breeze.

Once you have built up sufficient endurance, your aerobic sessions should last a minimum of about twenty minutes. It is believed to take approximately this long before fat is optimally released from cells and becomes available to be used as fuel. On the other hand, there are diminishing returns to performing cardio for extended periods of time. Lengthy, drawn-out aerobic sessions take a toll on your body and can easily lead to overtraining. Thus, to avoid any negative consequences, limit your sessions to no more than 45 minutes in length. By keeping the duration of your sessions between these prescribed boundaries, you'll maximize fat burning while mitigating any potential downside risk.

Intensity

Intensity is the key determinant in burning fat. There is a direct correlation between physical effort and caloric expenditure; the harder you work, the more calories you expend.

Some fitness professionals have perpetrated the myth that, for optimal fat burning, aerobics should be performed at a low level of intensity. This theory is predicated on the fact that a greater proportion of fat is burned during low-intensity exercise as opposed to exercise done at a higher level of intensity. However, the selective use of fat for fuel doesn't necessarily translate into a greater amount of fat loss. The loss of bodyfat is contingent on the total amount of fat calories burned—not the percentage of calories derived from fat—and, from this standpoint, high-intensity exercise invariably comes out ahead.

For example, if you burn 200 calories in a half hour by walking on the treadmill at a low level of intensity, approximately 60 percent of these calories will come from fat, giving you a net fat loss of 120 calories. On the other hand, exercising for the same amount of time at a high intensity will burn approximately 400 calories, with 160 of these calories coming from fat (even though the percentage of calories derived from fat is only 40 percent). Thus, if fat burning is your aim, performing cardiovascular exercise at a high level of intensity is clearly your best bet.

But how do you go about quantifying aerobic intensity? Commonly, women gauge their effort based on perspiration. The more they sweat, the harder they think they're working. However, while sweat often is associated with rigorous exercise, it actually is a poor indicator of intensity. When you exercise, sweat is brought on by an elevation of your body temperature. Your body regulates its temperature by activating your sweat glands, which then release water through your pores as a cooling mechanism. Hence, sweat is an indicator that your body temperature is rising, not necessarily that you are exercising at an intense level.

While there are many viable ways to gauge aerobic intensity, one of the easiest and most effective methods is by exercising in your target training zone. Your target training zone is based on a percentage of your age-related maximal heart rate. It can be determined by subtracting your age from 220 and then multiplying by the desired training intensity percentage. For example, if you are 20 years old and want to train at 80 percent intensity, your target heart rate would be 160 beats per minute ($220 - 20 = 200 \times .8 = 160$).

As a rule, your target training zone should be somewhere between 50 to 85 percent of your maximal heart rate. Keep your pace stable, beginning with a brief warm-up and finishing with a light cool-down. Every few minutes, check your pulse to make sure that you are maintaining your target zone. If your cardiovascular conditioning is poor, start out on the low end of the spectrum and gradually increase your intensity in increments of approximately 5 percent per week. It may take a while before you are able to maintain a high-intensity level; just be patient and it will happen.

WHAT'S THE BEST TIME TO EXERCISE?

In theory, it is best to perform aerobics first thing in the morning, on an empty stomach. The absence of food brings about a reduction in circulating blood sugar, causing glucose levels to fall. With a diminished availability of glucose, your body tends to rely more on fat to fuel your workout. Thus, from a fat-burning perspective, a case can be made for doing your cardio as soon as you roll out of bed.

However, not everyone functions well first thing in the morning. If you're more of a night bird, chances are that you'll sleepwalk through a morning workout. You'll have trouble generating sufficient intensity during training, resulting in poor exercise performance.

Therefore, in reality, the best time to exercise is when you are at your best. If you are a morning person, go ahead and train early. But if you don't really get going until you've been awake for several hours, by all means train later in the day. In the final analysis, let your biorhythms determine when you should work out.

Modalities

Consumers are forever searching for the "ultimate" cardiovascular activity, one that will literally melt away fat. Equipment manufacturers play into this mania. They are continuously flooding the market with new products, each promising to be the "premier fat-burning machine."

However, despite the hype, physiology dictates that no single activity can maximize your ability to burn fat; there simply is no one *best* cardiovascular exercise. As you may recall, the human body readily adjusts to an external stimulus by becoming more proficient. Hence, when the same exercise is used on a repeated basis, adaptation takes place, ultimately leading to diminished returns.

Only by cross training between different modalities can you prevent adaptation and thereby expedite the loss of bodyfat. Cross training is best accomplished by choosing several different activities and alternating them from one workout to the next. Not only does this constantly keep your body "offguard," but it also helps to reduce the likelihood of a training-related injury. Since each modality uses different muscles in exercise performance, your bones, muscles, and joints aren't subjected to continual impact. Accordingly, there is less wear and tear on your body, saving your musculoskeletal system from overuse.

Generally speaking, you are better off performing individual aerobic modalities rather than participating in group-based classes. Without question, aerobic classes can be fun. They provide a festive atmosphere, with lively music and dance-oriented maneuvers. They also can be a great place to socialize and meet new people, adding to the experience. For those who are not internally motivated to exercise, these factors can provide an impetus to become more active.

However, group-oriented activities have several drawbacks. First, by catering to the masses, it is unlikely that a class will specifically target your own heart rate. Second, because of the extreme, unorthodox nature of the movements involved, the risk of sustaining an injury is much greater in a class setting. So if you're looking for optimal results, group classes really aren't the best way to go.

Alternatively, individual aerobic modalities provide you with the ability to train within your target zone. Therefore, you can customize a routine to meet your specific needs, maximizing your fat-burning potential. And since individual modalities are executed in a controlled fashion, they tend to be much safer to perform.

So which aerobic modalities should you employ? In general, it makes sense to choose exercises that you enjoy. Theoretically, if you relish an activity, you'll be more likely keep up with your routine. However, try to keep an open mind and experiment with as many different activities as possible. The majority of exercise modalities allow you to read, watch television, and/or listen to music while you train. These diversions can make even the most mundane activity seem tolerable. Remember, variety is the spice of exercise—keep an open mind.

THE Q-ANGLE

Due to an increased Q-angle (the angle formed between the knee and hip), women are predisposed to knee-related injuries. Since women tend to have naturally wide hips (to accommodate the demands of childbirth), they generally have a larger Q-angle than their male counterparts. A large Q-angle causes lateral displacement of the femur (thighbone), heightening patellar forces during impact activities. As a rule, the wider your hips, the greater the risk of injury.

Although a regimented strength-training program will help to improve knee stability, care should be taken to ensure proper safety. Repeated use of high-impact maneuvers should be avoided. If clinically indicated, a neoprene brace can be utilized to provide greater stabilization to the area.

The following is an overview of the five most popular pieces of aerobic equipment. These machines can be found in virtually any gym and also are available to purchase for home use. It is important to note, however, that the equipment quality can vary significantly. If you choose to buy, make sure to shop around and try out a number of different units.

➡ ***Treadmill:*** The treadmill is probably the most widespread aerobic apparatus. It can be used to walk, jog, or run—or any combination of the three. The more expensive units have such features as preprogrammed workouts, built-in heart rate monitors, adjustable inclines, and others.

There are those who eschew the treadmill, preferring to run in the park or the street. Exercising in the great outdoors allows you to get some fresh air and sunshine and provides a sense of being in touch with nature. These are powerful allures for making aerobics more enjoyable.

However, the potential hazards of outdoor running can outweigh the benefits. When you run, a tremendous amount of downward force is exerted on your lower extremities. Each stride results in joint compression forces of up to 33 times bodyweight. For example, a 130-pound woman can conceivably put more than 4200 pounds of downward pressure on her joints each time her heel strikes the ground! Wet leaves, potholes, and other obstacles exacerbate the associated risks. This is why 70 percent of those who run on a frequent basis experience an injury to their lower extremities at some point in their lives.

The treadmill helps to mitigate these dangers. Since a treadmill has a cushioned surface, it absorbs some of the impact to your shins and knees. Consequently, the risk of injury to your lower extremities is significantly reduced.

HAND WEIGHTS AND THE TREADMILL

By holding onto hand weights while walking, you can substantially increase the amount of calories expended. This is an excellent way to burn additional fat while alleviating the wear and tear to the lower extremities. In fact, walking at 4 miles per hour with hand weights burns the same amount of calories as running at 5 miles per hour, with a 50 percent decrease in compression forces!

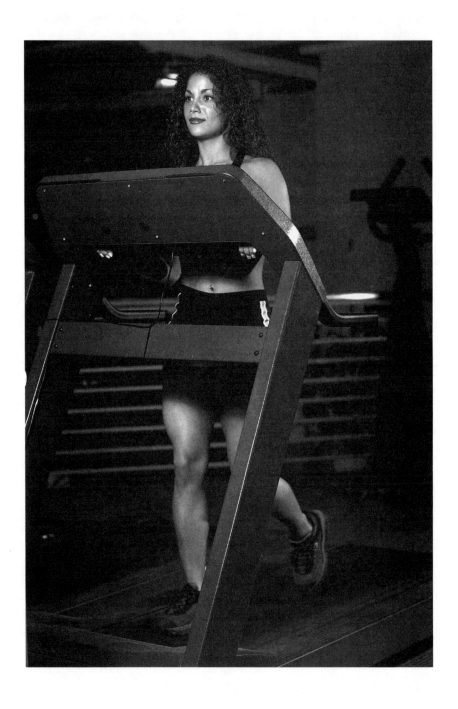

➡ ***Stationary Bike:*** Along with the treadmill, the stationary bike is an aerobic favorite. There are two basic types of bikes: upright and recumbent. Of the two, the recumbent is the decidedly better choice. It has an ergonomically designed seat that provides support for your back. This reduces stress to the lower lumbar region. The upright bike, on the other hand, has no such support. Hence, there is a tendency to lean forward during exercise, which can increase the potential for lower back injury.

Before using a bike, make sure to adjust the seat so that it corresponds to your height. Ideally, there should be a slight bend to your knees in the fully extended position. If your knees lock out, damage can occur to your connective tissue. Conversely, too much of a bend tends to overstretch the joint, which can also lead to injury.

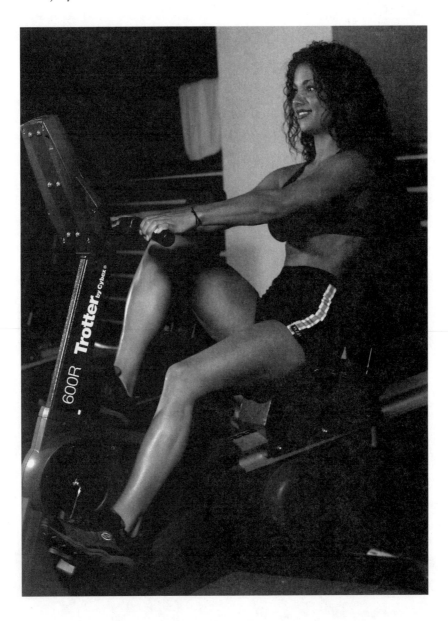

➠ ***Stair Climber:*** The stair climber (also called a stair stepper) is a mechanical version of, well, you guessed it, climbing stairs. Large pedals move in an up-and-down fashion, simulating the stair climbing motion. When proper intensity is utilized, this can provide a terrific cardiovascular workout.

Unfortunately, some women avoid the stair climber, believing that it increases the size of their butt. Rest assured, nothing can be further from the truth. The fact is, it's virtually impossible to increase muscle mass significantly through the performance of *any* endurance-related cardiovascular activity. The reason for this is simple: Aerobic exercise relies predominantly on slow-twitch muscle fibers during performance, with little activation of fast-twitch fibers. If you remember, fast-twitch fibers are the only type of fibers that have the ability to increase in size substantially. Since the stairmaster is aerobic in nature and therefore doesn't sufficiently activate fast-twitch fibers, it stands to reason that it can't contribute to building a substantial amount of muscle tissue in any part of the body, including your butt!

During performance, it is important to keep an upright posture; don't lean forward while stepping. Doing so places an inordinate amount of stress on the lumbar area, which easily can lead to lower back pain. Rather, maintain a slight lordotic curve (arched lower back), keeping your head up and chest out.

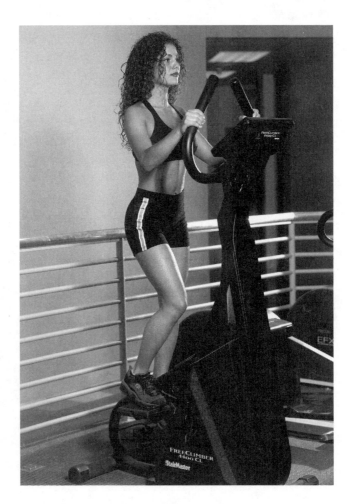

➡ ***Elliptical Trainer:*** The elliptical trainer is fast becoming a favorite in many gyms. Its sleek, space-aged design is an instant allure and its unique motion creates the feel of "moonwalking."

From a practical standpoint, the main advantage of the elliptical trainer is that it tends to reduce stress to the lower extremities. Its fluid, nonimpact motion tends to be easier on the joints, which can be particularly beneficial for those who have existing injuries to the hips, knees, or ankles.

During performance, you have the choice of pedaling in either a forward or backward direction. It is best to employ both options. This allows different muscle fibers to be recruited, providing more complete aerobic conditioning.

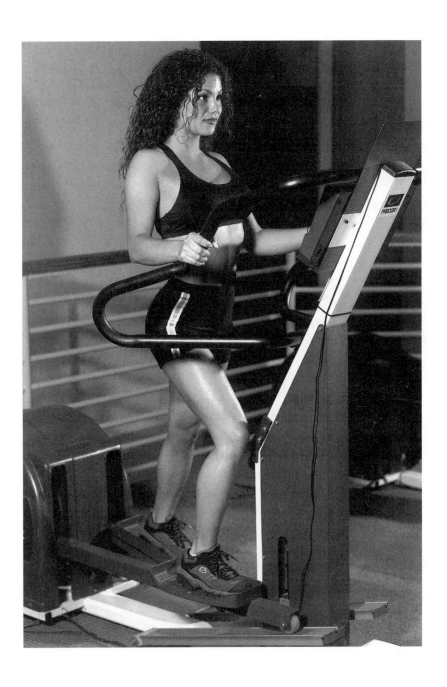

➠ *Rowing Machine:* The rowing machine is perhaps the most underutilized of all the cardiovascular modalities. With all the new aerobic devices on the market, the rowing machine basically has been relegated to second-tier status. Yet rowing is one of the best ways to condition the upper body—something lacking in most aerobic activities.

Contrary to popular belief, upper body aerobics promote a greater caloric expenditure when compared with activities that are limited to the lower body. This is largely attributable to the metabolic cost of stabilizer muscles that are recruited to support the torso when the arms are aerobically trained. Hence, aerobic exercise that involves the upper body actually is a very efficient means for expediting the loss of body fat. What's more, since cardiovascular benefits are specific to the muscles being worked, additional aerobic pathways (i.e., enzymes, mitochondria, capillaries, etc.) are established in the upper body, helping to expedite fat burning.

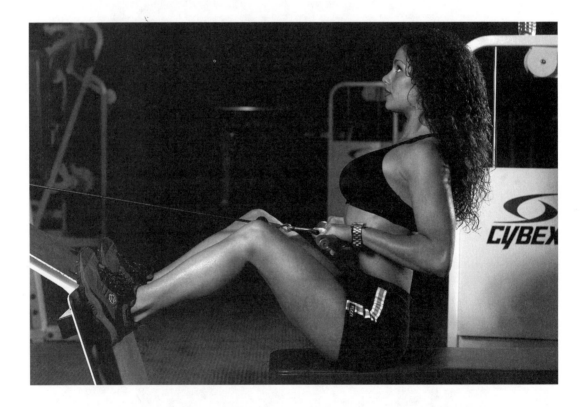

It must be noted, however, that upper body aerobics tend to elevate blood pressure during training. Because the circulatory capacity is lower in the arms than in the legs, there is an increased resistance to blood flow in this region, which, in turn, causes blood pressure to rise. Accordingly, for those with existing hypertension of cardiovascular disease, upper body aerobics may be contraindicated.

Of course, there are many other activities that make fine aerobic choices. Ballroom dancing, rollerblading, cross country skiing—the list goes on and on. But regardless of which activities you choose to employ, make sure you are training with sufficient intensity to generate results. You'd need to play several hours of doubles tennis, for example, in order to burn the same amount of calories in a half-hour run!

Table 8.1 summarizes the High-Energy Fitness™ protocols for cardiovascular training. As with weight training, proper manipulation of these protocols will determine how far you will ultimately excel in your efforts. Since your aerobic routine will impact on your weight-training program, striking the right balance between the two is essential in optimizing your physique. It is advisable to proceed cautiously here, starting with the minimum recommended levels and advancing with care. While the usual inclination is to go all out, you run the risk of pushing the envelope too far. As with most things in life, discretion is the better part of valor.

TABLE 8.1

Duration	Frequency	Intensity	Modalities
20 to 45 minutes per session	3 to 5 days a week	50% to 85% of maximal heart rate, progressively increasing intensity over time	Alternate between as many different modalities as possible

EAT TO LOSE

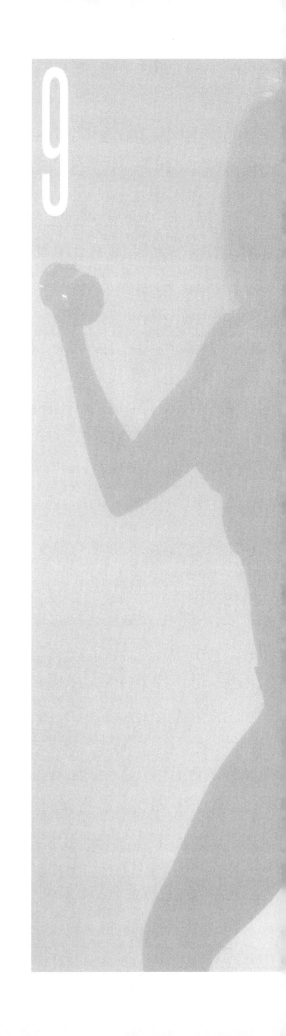

Virtually every woman is, at one time or another, on a diet. Slim is in, and women are willing to try virtually anything in order to win the battle of the bulge. There are high-carb/low-fat diets, low-carb/high-fat diets, all-fruit diets, no-fruit diets, and even cabbage soup diets! From Atkins to the Zone, diets span the alphabet from A to Z.

However, the stark reality is that diets don't work! While most of these programs will induce temporary weight loss, they simply don't provide the ability to sustain this weight loss over the long haul. They are short-term solutions to a long-term problem and neglect to teach a woman proper eating patterns. Sadly, only 10 percent of those who go on a diet are able to keep the weight off after a year's time.

Worse yet, repeated cycles of weight loss and regain (called yo-yo dieting) can severely suppress metabolism and cause a rebound effect. During each diet cycle, the body continually trains itself to survive on fewer and fewer calories. Hence, it becomes increasingly more difficult to shed unwanted pounds and, in the end, regained weight is almost always higher than it was before dieting.

Actually, when applied to weight loss, the term *diet* is a misnomer. If you look in the dictionary, a diet is defined as "food and drink regularly provided or consumed." It is a normal meal plan that provides habitual nourishment—not a quick means to lose weight. Thus, from here on, the term *diet* will be used in the context of its intended meaning—to describe a regimented program of eating.

It is important to realize that there is no single "best" diet. Every woman has a unique nutritional profile and will respond differently to various foods based on a host of genetic and lifestyle factors. Things such as metabolic rate, insulin sensitivity, and activity level all influence dietary requirements. Therefore, you can't simply follow a cookie-cutter nutritional prescription and expect it to work for you. Chances are, your specific needs won't be adequately addressed.

The key to promoting long-term, sustainable weight management is to develop a sound nutritional strategy that becomes a way of life. An effective program balances caloric intake with caloric expenditure, stabilizes insulin, and increases metabolism. It must be sensible as well as practical. My approach to nutrition combines all of these facets. The program that I espouse is based on nutritional science—not gimmickry. It is specific in its recommendations, yet it is flexible enough to be adapted to your individual needs. Whether you want to lose, gain, or maintain your current weight, this program will help you achieve your goals.

Before discussing which foods to eat, you need to determine your caloric intake. Calories *do* count and, despite the claims of some so-called nutritional "experts," the amount of food that you ingest will have a major impact on whether weight is gained or lost.

The first step in determining caloric intake is to figure out your daily caloric maintenance level (DCML): the number of calories required each day to maintain a stable body weight. A simple way to estimate DCML is to multiply your bodyweight by 12 (bodyweight X 12). Thus, a woman who weighs 120 pounds would need approximately 1440 calories to maintain her current weight. While this formula only provides a crude approximation of daily caloric intake, it at least gives you a starting point from which to work. From here, modifications can be made based on individual requirements.

If weight loss is desired, your DCML must be adjusted so you expend more calories than you consume. This is simple mathematics. You can eat all the "right" foods, but if you take in too many calories from these foods, weight gain is inevitable. For example, consuming as few as 100 extra calories a day—the amount found in a handful of nachos or a dozen french fries—can result in a yearly weight gain of more than 10 pounds! Only by creating a caloric deficit is weight loss possible.

For safe, effective weight loss, a maximum of 1 to 2 pounds can be lost per week. Don't be lured in by unscrupulous ads that promise to take off 30 pounds in thirty days. These quick-fix programs are unhealthy and counterproductive. When calories are severely restricted, up to 45 percent of the energy deficit is derived from burning muscle tissue for fuel. This can account for as much as 1 pound a week of muscle loss. As previously discussed, muscle is highly metabolic. It speeds up resting metabolic rate and thereby accelerates the body's ability to burn fat. Thus, by depleting muscle tissue, fat burning is inhibited, inevitably leading to an increase in bodyfat.

Your best bet is to take it slow. A loss of 1 pound per week might not seem like a lot on the surface but, over the course of a year, it equates to a 50-pound drop! Start out with a 300-calorie reduction in your DCML and then gradually increase this amount if necessary. But don't go overboard! Remember, rapid weight loss will sabotage your long-term fitness goals. If you experience a loss of more than 2 pounds in a week, increase caloric intake accordingly to stay in the prescribed range.

Initially, it can be helpful to weigh your food on a scale. A digital food scale is relatively inexpensive and easy to use. While this may seem like a chore, it really is worth the effort. Weighing your food takes only a few seconds and requires no clean-up. Within a short period of time, you'll develop a sense of how much to eat and soon will be able to estimate portion sizes on your own.

Once you have determined your caloric intake, you must now focus on the percentage of calories that will be derived from carbohydrates, protein, and fat—the so-called macronutrients. To get the most out of your diet, it is imperative that you take in the right mix of these nutrients. Those who believe the old adage that "a calorie is a calorie" are sadly mistaken. Each nutrient has specific functions and affects the body in different ways. Let's discuss how these nutrients should be apportioned for optimal benefits.

Carbohydrates

For those who are trying to stay lean, carbs can be a double-edged sword. On one hand, carbs are the body's preferred source of metabolic energy. They help to preserve tissue proteins, assist in fat metabolism, and stoke the central nervous system.

Carbs are particularly important as you exercise. The compounds derived from carbohydrate breakdown are stored as glycogen in your muscles and liver. Glycogen is the primary fuel used to power your muscles during intense workouts. It provides an instant source of energy that can be accessed on demand, enabling you to train in an all-out fashion.

When carbohydrates are severely restricted in the diet, your body has to covert amino acids into glucose (through a process called gluconeogenesis) in order to meet short-term energy needs. However, this conversion process is very inefficient and fails to supply adequate energy reserves. Ultimately, your stamina begins to wane and you soon become lethargic and irritable. Complications including nausea, headaches, and dizziness are apt to occur. There is a degradation in exercise performance, diminishing your capacity to generate lean muscle tone. Overall, your ability to function at a high level is seriously impaired.

On the other hand, carbs trigger the release of insulin in the body. When ingested, carbs are broken down into simple sugars. In turn, the pancreas must secrete insulin to clear the surplus sugar from the bloodstream. However, while insulin plays an important role in regulating body function, it also can be detrimental to weight management. You see, insulin is a storage hormone that is directly responsible for converting sugars into bodyfat as well as inhibiting the conversion of stored fat into energy. This double whammy greatly increases the potential for bodyfat storage.

Because of this effect on insulin, it is essential to regulate the types and amount of carbohydrates for optimal weight management. Make no mistake: All carbs are not created equal! Although most people know that it's important to cut back on fatty foods, they often are oblivious to the types of carbohydrates in their diet.

A common way to distinguish carbs is by their complexity. You've probably heard about the differences between "simple" and "complex" carbs. However, a better mode of classification is based on the glycemic index. The glycemic index provides a more accurate indication of how carbs affect insulin secretion. Carbs that cause a rapid elevation of blood sugar (glucose) are termed high glycemic, while those that are "time released" and maintain stable levels of blood sugar are called low glycemic.

High-glycemic carbs tend to have a negative impact on your physique. The problem with these foods is that they are rapidly assimilated, causing a spike in your blood-sugar levels. Consequently, a large quantity of insulin is needed to stabilize blood sugar. This increased insulin production turns on fat storage mechanisms and blocks certain enzymes that are responsible for lipolysis (fat breakdown). Ultimately, excess nutrients are shuttled into adipose cells, resulting in a corresponding increase in bodyfat.

Furthermore, this rush of insulin clears sugars from your circulatory system in such an expeditious fashion that it creates a rebound effect, producing a sudden and dramatic drop in blood sugar levels. A hypoglycemic state is induced, causing severe hunger pangs and food cravings. This creates a vicious cycle that encourages you to binge out on high-glycemic foods. As a result, more calories are consumed and fat storage is heightened even further.

Conversely, low-glycemic foods are broken down more slowly. They enter the bloodstream in a time-released fashion, keeping blood sugar levels in check. Insulin, therefore, is released gradually into your system. Stable insulin levels mean reduced bodyfat storage. And, because there's a steady stream of glucose, your energy levels remain high.

Hence, if you want to stay lean, keep your consumption of high-glycemic foods—especially refined sugars—to an absolute minimum. When eaten in abundance, they can be one of the biggest obstacles to maintaining a lean physique—perhaps even more so than foods laden with fat. Remember: Just because a food is "fat free" doesn't mean it won't make you fat—it also must be low glycemic to qualify as a healthy choice. Accordingly, stay away from such high-glycemic choices as sweetened cereals, potatoes, white rice, and white flour breads. Instead, replace them with oatmeal, yams, brown rice, and whole grains. If you do choose to consume a high-glycemic food, make sure you eat it in conjunction with a protein-based source. This will help to slow down absorption and mitigate its effect on insulin secretions.

Fiber is another important component of carbohydrate intake. There is a large body of scientific evidence indicating that a diet high in fiber is beneficial to your health. At the very least, fiber helps to maintain bowel regularity. Because fiber absorbs water in the large intestine, it causes your stools to become soft and fluffy, thereby preventing constipation. The increase in stool volume also helps to dilute the concentration of bile acids, which are thought to instigate the growth of malignant tumors. Studies have shown up to a 30 percent reduction in these malignancies, making fiber a potent cancer-fighting agent.

In addition, fiber consumption can cause a substantial decline in serum cholesterol levels. Reductions of up to 13 percent have been reported, with favorable effects on the ratio of "good" to "bad" cholesterol (HDL to LDL). Since each 1 percent drop in cholesterol translates into a 2 percent drop in the risk of developing heart disease, the cardioprotective effects of fiber are far reaching.

Besides having a positive effect on your well-being, fiber also plays an important role in weight management. By forming a "gel" in the intestines, it inhibits the digestion and absorption of nutrients. As food passes through your intestines, some of the nutrients get trapped in the gel and end up being excreted before they can be metabolized. Hence, you can eat more food without having it stored in your system. In fact, it has been reported that, by simply doubling fiber intake from 18 to 36 grams, you reduce the available calories in your diet by more than 100 calories per day!

Fiber is found in a wide array of carb-based foods. Appendix A shows some of the more popular high-fiber foods as well as their corresponding fiber content. Consume them readily. By maintaining a high-fiber diet, you'll go a long way to improving your health as well as your body.

Recommended Intake: Carbs should comprise approximately 40 to 50 percent of the calories in your diet. This will sufficiently replenish glycogen reserves without having an adverse effect on insulin levels. Start out on the low end of the spectrum, keeping carbs at the suggested minimum. If you feel lethargic or fatigued, increase carbs another 5 percent. If you still don't have enough energy, take carbs up to the maximum.

Green vegetables should make up a healthy portion of carb intake. On a volume basis, they are extremely low in calories and high in nutritional value. Think of them as green water—they can be consumed in large amounts without making you fat. A pound of broccoli, for instance, contains only about 120 calories (compare that to a pound of pasta, which has about 1600 calories!). Moreover, because of their bulk, green vegetables take up a large amount of space in the stomach. This helps to suppress food cravings, thereby preventing the urge to overeat. And considering that they are replete with vitamins and minerals, green vegetables should be a staple in your diet.

Protein

Without question, protein is the king of all nutrients. It provides the building blocks for enzymes and hormones, enables nerve and brain cells to communicate effectively with one another, and fosters the repair and growth of muscle tissue. Every cell in your body contains protein; life could not go on without it.

A diet high in protein has a multitude of benefits. First, protein has a greater thermic effect than any other nutrient. Because of its chemical structure, a great deal of energy is expended in the breakdown of protein. Up to 25 percent of protein-based calories are burned in this process. Of course, with fewer calories available for storage, the potential for weight gain is diminished.

Protein also is the most satisfying of all the macronutrients. On a calorie-for-calorie basis, protein fills you up more than either carbs or fat. This is largely due to the secretion of satiety hormones, especially cholecystokinin (CCK). Studies have shown that when people consume a calorie-restricted diet consisting of carbs, protein, or fat, only those on the protein diet demonstrate a significant reduction in hunger sensation. Similar findings have been shown for caloric intake; people following a protein-based diet tend to eat significantly fewer calories than those on a carb- or fat-based diet. The evidence is clear: When protein consumption is high, you're less inclined to binge out on large meals.

In addition, adequate protein is necessary to remain in positive nitrogen balance, a condition that prevents the breakdown of muscle tissue and accelerates recuperation from exercise. When protein intake is insufficient, nitrogen is excreted at a greater rate than it's consumed, sending your body into a catabolic state. Overtraining is likely to occur and muscular development suffers.

Furthermore, as opposed to carbohydrates, protein has a negligible effect on insulin levels. Protein is not directly broken down into glucose. It must first undergo a complex conversion process called *deamination* before it can be assimilated and synthesized by the body. This helps to keep blood sugar in check, preventing the oversecretion of insulin. Moreover, protein tends to increase the production of glucagon, a hormone that opposes the effect of insulin. Since a primary function of glucagon is to signal the body to burn fat for fuel, fat loss, rather than fat gain, is promoted.

There is a widespread fallacy that high-protein diets are harmful to your health. This myth is based on the contention that a surplus of protein has a detrimental effect on kidney function. Undeniably, the digestion of protein results in the accretion of urea, a byproduct of amino acid breakdown. In theory, a large buildup of urea overtaxes the kidneys and impairs their ability to function. However, as long as you don't have existing renal disease, your kidneys are more than able to handle this overload. Provided you take in a sufficient quantity of fluids, any excess urea will be readily excreted from your body with no ill effect on renal function.

Recommended Intake: Protein should account for 30 to 40 percent of total calories, equating to roughly 1 to 1.25 grams of protein per pound of bodyweight. Hence, a woman weighing 120 pounds needs to consume a minimum of 120 grams of protein per day. Any less and you risk falling into a negative nitrogen balance. Disregard the United States Department of Agriculture (USDA) recommended daily allowance (RDA) for protein (an absurdly low 4/10 of a gram per pound of bodyweight). The RDA is based on the needs of sedentary people and doesn't take into account the increased demand required for active individuals.

Make sure that your choice of proteins comes from lean sources. Skinless poultry breast, lean red meats, seafood, and egg whites are excellent choices. For convenience, there are a wide variety of protein powders available at health stores and other outlets. Whey protein powders are generally your best choice, followed by egg, casein, and vegetable sources.

Fat

Traditional wisdom has always been that if you want to maintain a lean physique, dietary fat should be kept to a bare minimum. For many years, the majority of sports nutritionists emphatically stated, "Eat fat and you'll get fat!" A legion of health-conscious consumers listened, and zero-fat diets soon became the rage. The prevailing sentiment was to cut out every last gram of fat from a diet. More recently, this view has softened, and certain classifications of fat are now being recommended as part of one's daily diet.

Certainly, fats are an essential nutrient and play a vital role in many bodily functions. They are involved in cushioning your internal organs for protection, aiding in the absorption of vitamins, and facilitating the production of cell membranes, hormones, and prostaglandins. Physiologically, it would be impossible to survive without the inclusion of fats in your diet.

Fats are classified into two basic categories: saturated and unsaturated. Saturated fats are abundant in many meats, oils, and dairy products. They are biologically inert, having no functional utility. After consumption, they either are stored in adipose cells throughout your body or become oxidized as fatty deposits in your arteries. Over time, your arteries narrow, resulting in severe atherosclerosis—a direct precursor to a heart attack. But that's not all. These fats tend to make your muscles less responsive to insulin and inhibit your body's ability to store sugars as glycogen. Studies have shown that the consumption of saturated fat is directly correlated with fat storage: The more you eat, the more you keep. Therefore, you must keep your consumption of saturated fats to an absolute minimum. Eliminate them at all costs.

Alternatively, unsaturated fats are healthier fats. In particular, specific types of unsaturated fats, called essential fatty acids (EFAs), are especially beneficial. EFAs cannot be manufactured by your body and hence, like vitamins, are an "essential" component in food. Due to their lack of saturation, they don't readily bond together (that's why they remain liquid at room temperature) and therefore can be synthesized for systemic use. In addition, they are extremely biologically active and help to increase your metabolic rate while enhancing the ability of your muscles to use insulin. Ultimately, this results in better fat metabolism and improved body composition.

The best sources of EFAs are found in soy products and deep-colored, cold-water fish such as salmon, mackerel, and tuna. Flaxseed oil also contains high levels of EFAs. It comes in liquid form and either can be mixed into your foods or taken by the spoonful. Look for a brand that has a 3 : 1 ratio of omega-3 (linolenic acid) to omega-6 EFAs (linoleic acid).

> **TIPS FOR REDUCING SATURATED FATS**
>
> 1. **Foods should be baked, broiled, steamed, or microwaved. Never deep fry foods.**
> 2. **Prepare your foods "dry," without using lard, oil, or butter in your cooking**
> 3. **Trim all visible fat from your meats. Even lean cuts of meat normally have fat around the edges. Any fat that can be seen by the naked eye should be removed.**
> 4. **Remove the skin from poultry products. Do this *before* cooking since heat causes animal fat to seep into the meat.**

Recommended Intake: As a rule, limit your fat intake to no more than 20 percent of your total calories, with the majority coming from EFAs. Despite the recent prominence of high-fat diets, excess fat consumption will almost certainly have a negative long-term impact on your physique. Since virtually no energy is expended in their digestion, fats are more easily stored as bodyfat than any other nutrient. While proteins and carbs have a thermic effect on the body, the percentage of calories expended in the breakdown of fat is minimal.

Moreover, fats are calorically dense. Each gram of fat has nine calories, as compared to carbohydrates and protein, which have only four. Hence, a small portion of a fat-laden food has a much higher amount of calories than a comparable portion of a low-fat food. For example, a sliver of chocolate cake might contain 200 calories, while it would take about 2 pounds of green beans to equal this amount! Since it takes a large quantity of fatty foods to sate the stomach, the potential for overeating is dramatically increased.

Thus, don't buy into the high-fat hype. Eat only enough to fulfill your basic requirements. If you want to look great naked, lower fat is definitely the way to go.

Putting It All Together

Table 9.1 summarizes the nutritional protocols that will help you look great naked. Use these protocols as a guideline and adopt them to your individual needs. As previously stated, every woman is unique. Hence, there is no one best nutritional program. Experiment with different nutrient ratios and see how it affects your body. Over time, you'll find out what works best for you.

TABLE 9.1

Nutrient	Recommended Percentage of Total Calories	Specific Recommendations
Carbohydrates	40 to 50%	• Eat low-glycemic carbs • Take in a high amount of fiber
Protein	30 to 40%	• Eat lean, high-quality protein sources
Fat	15 to 20%	• Eat mostly unsaturated, essential fatty acids

SHED THOSE LAST FEW POUNDS

The complexities of nutrition go beyond carbs, protein, and fat. While there's little doubt that the amount and proportion of these macronutrients are the dominant factors in weight management, other nutritional aspects can have a significant impact on your physique, too.

The following eight strategies will help to elevate your metabolism and maximize your body's fat-burning ability. By integrating these principles into your nutritional approach, it's possible to achieve a leaner physique without altering caloric intake. This is especially pertinent when it comes to shedding those last few pounds which always seem so hard to get rid of.

Eat Small, Frequent Meals

In today's fast-paced world, most women give little thought about the timing of their meals. All too often, breakfast consists only of a cup of coffee. Succeeding meals are eaten whenever there is a free moment, usually culminating with a large feast at dinner and possibly a midnight snack.

Unfortunately, this type of nutritional regimen has a deleterious effect on your body composition. When you deprive your body of food for more than a few hours, it senses that it won't have adequate fuel to carry out daily activities and shifts into a "starvation mode" as a means of conserving energy. Consequently, your metabolic rate slows down, preventing additional burning of calories. The end result is an increase in bodyfat levels with a corresponding loss of lean muscle tissue.

By regimenting your eating patterns and consuming small, frequent meals, your body is able to operate at peak efficiency. Nutrients are better absorbed into your system, allowing them to be efficiently utilized for important biological functions. Your metabolism revs up, increasing your body's internal production of heat (a process called thermogenesis), which, in turn, helps to burn fat for fuel. Moreover, your appetite remains suppressed, making you less likely to binge out on a big meal late in the day.

There also is an expenditure of energy in the digestion process, called dietary-induced thermogenesis. Every time you eat, your body burns off approximately 10 percent of the calories consumed, keeping your metabolism elevated for up to several hours after consumption. By constantly taking in food, you increase dietary-induced thermogenesis and thus maintain a raised metabolic rate throughout the day.

Ideally, you should space out your meals evenly, eating five or six times a day at regular intervals. While this might seem like a time-consuming chore, it actually can be accomplished without a great deal of effort. For instance, you can prepare several meals in advance, store them in plastic containers, and reheat them in a microwave on an as-needed basis. As an alternative, you can supplement your basic meals with powdered meal replacements or sports bars. These "engineered foods" provide the ultimate in convenience: They are nutritionally balanced, easily transportable, and can be prepared in a matter of minutes.

Decrease Starchy Carbs at Night

For most women, starchy carbs make up a substantial portion of their evening meals. Pasta, rice, potatoes . . . these are nightly staples in the standard American diet. Steak and fries, spaghetti and meatballs—what would dinner be without them?

The trouble with starchy carbs is that they are readily transformed to fat when eaten before bedtime. The reason for this is simple: The primary function of carbohydrates is to supply short-term energy for your daily activities. If carbs are not used immediately for fuel, they have two possible fates: They either are stored as glycogen in your liver and muscles or are converted into fatty acids and stored in adipose tissue as bodyfat. Since activity levels usually are lowest during the evening hours, there is a diminished use of carbs for fuel and therefore an increased potential for bodyfat storage.

In general, the best time to consume carbs is early in the day, when your activity levels are at their peak. This will allow your body to utilize a maximal amount of carbs for energy and minimize the potential for fat deposition. Breakfast, in particular, is an excellent time to load up on complex carbs. A large bowl of rolled oats or bran cereal will set the stage for fueling your daily activities and keep you physically and mentally fit throughout the day.

On the other hand, it is best to limit your dinner fare to fibrous, vegetable-based carbohydrate sources. Fibrous vegetables tend to be extremely low in total calories and, because of their bulk, are very filling. For supper, consider eating a meal consisting of lean poultry or fish combined with a large bowl of salad greens. Other vegetables, such as broccoli, string beans, cauliflower, and zucchini, also make fine nighttime carbohydrate choices and will reduce the potential for unwanted bodyfat storage.

Stay Hydrated

Believe it or not, most of your body is made up of water. Your muscles are roughly 75 percent water, your blood is more than 80 percent water and your lungs are almost 90 percent water. Clearly, water is the most vital of all nutrients—without it, you would die in a matter of days.

Regrettably, some women cut back on their fluid intake, thinking that it will help to eliminate subcutaneous water retention. In some cases, they'll go so far as to refrain from drinking liquids altogether. What a big mistake! When fluids are restricted, your body senses a threat to its survival and tries to hold onto to every last drop of water. The end result is an increase in water retention, leaving you puffy and bloated.

Worse, fluid restriction tends to make you fatter. Without an adequate supply of water, your kidney function becomes impaired, causing a systemic accumulation of metabolic waste. Your liver, in turn, has to work overtime to flush out these toxins from your body. This compromises your liver's ability to metabolize fat into usable energy—one of its primary responsibilities. As a result, less fat is metabolized, causing an increase in adipose storage.

In order to avoid this fate, water should be readily consumed. Aim to drink at least at least a gallon of fluids daily, spacing out intake throughout the day. Alcohol-

and caffeine-based beverages don't count toward this amount; they have a diuretic effect and actually cause you to dehydrate. Rather, your best bet is to drink plain old water, and a lot of it. Although tap water will suffice, natural spring water is a decidedly better choice. It is devoid of the pollutants that taint our reservoirs and therefore keeps your body free of contaminants. If possible, the water should be chilled or served on ice. Cold water is absorbed into the system more quickly than warm water, ensuring a continued state of hydration.

During exercise, fluid intake should be increased still further. As you work out, a large amount of water is lost through your sweat, breath, and urine. If these fluids aren't replenished, your exercise performance is bound to suffer. In fact, a mere 3 percent reduction in water can cause up to a 10 percent loss in muscular strength. When taken to the extreme, heat stroke or even circulatory collapse can occur. Clearly, exercise-induced dehydration must be avoided at all costs.

It is a mistake, however, to rely on thirst as an indicator for to when to drink. Intense exercise inhibits the thirst sensors in your throat and gut; by the time you become thirsty, your body already is severely dehydrated. Therefore, during exercise, drink early and drink often. Consume 8 ounces of fluid immediately before your workout and then take small sips of water every five or ten minutes or so while training.

Jumpstart with Java

Caffeine has gotten a bad rap. For years, health care practitioners have denounced it as a health hazard. They've cautioned against its use, citing studies that link it to everything from heart disease to cancer. However, the bulk of these studies were flawed in their design. Some used enormous quantities of caffeine—far beyond what the normal individual consumes. Others employed insufficient sample sizes or had errors in statistical analysis. The truth is, when all the available information is examined, there's really no evidence that modest caffeine consumption causes any detriments to overall health and well-being. In fact, a few studies actually found a negative correlation between caffeine and certain forms of cancer!

Does this mean that you should load up on caffeinated beverages? Absolutely not! Caffeine is a stimulant. At high doses, it can cause a host of unwanted side-effects such as hypertension, nervousness, insomnia, and gastrointestinal distress. Guzzling mass quantities of coffee and cola will only serve to make you wired and irritable—not lean and defined.

However, when used in moderation, caffeine can be a safe and effective means of expediting a loss of bodyfat. By stimulating brown adipose tissue (BAT)—a special type of fat that elevates metabolism—caffeine facilitates the release of free fatty acids from adipocytes, allowing fat to be utilized for short-term energy. Studies have shown up to a 4 percent increase in resting metabolic rate from judicious caffeine supplementation, with effects lasting up to several hours after ingestion.

You don't need to take a lot of caffeine to derive positive benefits. A daily dose of 200 to 300 milligrams is all that's required to rev up your metabolic rate. Two cups of brewed coffee first thing in the morning will satisfy this requirement quite nicely. Better yet, consume the coffee immediately before your workout. In addition to its fat-burning effects, caffeine helps to delay fatigue and improve exercise intensity. Your performance will be enhanced, spurring you on to greater gains.

But remember to avoid going overboard with caffeine consumption. Excessive intake has no additional benefits and can actually impede results. When consumed in abundance, caffeine acts as a *vasoconstrictor*, narrowing arteries and restricting blood flow. As you may recall, a reduced circulatory capacity inhibits the breakdown of stored bodyfat. Ultimately, this counteracts the thermogenic effects of caffeine, nullifying its fat-burning benefits.

For best results, black coffee or espresso is recommended; the increased calories associated with adding cream or sugar will easily offset the caffeine-induced increase in metabolic rate. If black coffee is simply too bitter for your taste buds, then try using skim milk and/or artificial sweeteners as flavor enhancers.

Go Easy on the Sauce

The world floats on a sea of alcohol. Whether it's the two-martini lunch, the evening happy hour, or the after-dinner drink, alcohol is firmly ingrained in today's society. It is, without question, the most popular recreational drug in existence. In many circles, getting drunk even is a rite of passage—a rite that often continues throughout adulthood. With such widespread social acceptance, it's no wonder that approximately half of all Americans drink on a regular basis and more than 5 percent are heavy drinkers.

However, for any woman who aspires to maximize her body's potential, alcohol is a definite taboo. Make no mistake; alcohol will make you fat. It is calorically dense, containing over seven calories per gram (as opposed to carbs and protein, which have four). And this doesn't include the addition of mixers, which can significantly increase the calorie count. Take a look at the caloric content in some popular alcoholic beverages: A margarita has 600 calories, a martini 250, and a beer 150—pretty heavy stuff! What's more, these drinks are virtually devoid of any nutritional value. They are "empty calories" that do nothing but pack on unwanted pounds. Considering these facts, there is no doubt that even moderate drinking can have a decidedly negative impact on your figure.

Moreover, it is difficult for the body to break down alcohol. The liver must use a tremendous amount of coenzymes (such as NAD [nicotinamide adenine dinucleotide] and FAD [flavin adenine diinucleotide]) in order to assimilate the toxins from alcohol. Consequently, there are fewer coenzymes available to carry out vital metabolic functions, including the breakdown of fat for energy. The end result: increased fat storage. This process can begin after just a single night of heavy drinking.

With chronic abuse, the consequences of alcohol can be disastrous—often irreparable. Alcohol is a poison. It infiltrates your internal organs and has a toxic effect on everything that it comes into contact with. Your liver and spleen, in particular, become severely impaired and lose their ability to carry out vital functions. Forget about losing bodyfat; your entire metabolic system becomes dysfunctional. And don't think your muscles are immune from the carnage. Sustained bouts of heavy drinking ultimately cause myopathy—a degeneration of muscle tissue that obliterates your hard-earned gains.

The best advice on alcohol is to limit consumption to an absolute minimum; if possible, eliminate it completely from your diet. Get used to the idea that you don't need alcohol to have a good time. If you're out at a party or dance club, order a club soda with a twist of lemon or lime. Once you have adjusted to being a teetotaler, you'll soon appreciate the associated benefits. When others are in a drunken stupor, you'll be in full control of your faculties. You'll wake up hangover free, never having to regret what you did the night before. And, of course, you'll keep your body operating at peak efficiency, maintaining optimal shape year round.

Hold the Salt

Salt is the most widely used of all spices. It is added to almost every food imaginable, from soup to nuts and everything in between.

The craving for salt is physiologic. You see, there are distinct taste buds that are specifically receptive to salty foods. It is believed these taste buds reside on the tip and upper front portion of the tongue, producing a desire to consume salt.

Salt is comprised of sodium (as well as chloride), a basic mineral that's abundant in nature. Because it carries an electrical charge, sodium is considered an *electrolyte*. In conjunction with potassium, it is responsible for regulating the body's fluid balance; potassium maintains the fluid balance intracellularly (within the cells) while sodium maintains the balance of fluids extracellularly (outside of the cells). Hence, sodium is essential for bodily function; a lack of it leads to hyponatremia, a condition that ultimately causes death.

Although it is an essential nutrient, only minute quantities of sodium are required through dietary means. In fact, a mere 500 milligrams is all that's needed to maintain normal biological function—an amount that equates to about 1/4 of a teaspoon of salt. Yet the average American consumes more than ten times this quantity! When too much sodium is ingested, fluid is drawn out of the cells and into the body's free spaces, causing the malady known as water retention. Your feet and hands swell, your face becomes puffy, and water accumulates beneath your skin; not an enviable condition for someone trying to maintain a lean, toned physique. The fact is, sodium occurs naturally in most foods, and you'll get all you need just by eating a sensible diet.

The best way to avoid an overconsumption of sodium is by eating fresh, unprocessed foods. Stay away from all prepackaged and canned goods. They tend to be the worst offenders. Many condiments and sauces also are loaded with sodium. Ketchup, salad dressings, and soy sauce all contain whopping amounts. And in order to avoid any hidden sources, get used to reading food labels. The sodium content is plainly listed for all to see.

In addition, refrain from adding salt to your meals. If you want to spice up your foods, there are dozens of delicious seasonings that can enhance flavor without any side-effects. Paprika, cinnamon, basil, oregano, garlic—the list goes on. Experiment with different combinations and see what you find palatable. By using a little ingenuity, you can create tasty dishes that are virtually sodium free.

Have an Antioxidant Cocktail

Much has been made about vitamin and mineral supplementation. For many generations, these so-called micronutrients were touted as wonder supplements, heralded for curing everything from the common cold to night blindness. While we now know these claims to be greatly exaggerated, this doesn't diminish the fact that micronutrients are imperative for maintaining a fit, healthy body.

Vitamins and minerals serve many important biological functions. They facilitate energy transfer, prevent disease, and act as coenzymes to assist in many chemical reactions. A deficiency in any of these micronutrients can lead to severe illness. Don't worry, though. If you follow the nutritional recommendations outlined in this book, you'll more than meet your daily requirements.

There is, however, a special class of micronutrients called antioxidants, which are required in much larger amounts than other vitamins and minerals. Antioxidants are the body's scavengers. They help to defend the body against damage caused by free radicals—unstable molecules that can injure healthy cells and tissues. Millions of these dangerous villains are produced each day during the normal course of respiration. The main culprit is oxygen. Every time you breathe, oxygen uptake causes free radical production. Environmental factors such as pollutants, smoke, and certain chemicals also contribute to their formation. If left unchecked, free radicals can wreak havoc on your physique and cause a multitude of ailments, including arthritis, cardiovascular disease, dementia, and cancer.

For the active woman, antioxidants are of particular importance. Due to increased oxygen consumption, free radical production skyrockets during exercise. This results in an inflammation of muscle tissue, impairing muscular function and slowing recovery. The capacity for muscular repair is reduced, heightening the likelihood of overtraining.

Fortunately, like heroic warriors, antioxidants engulf free radicals, rendering them harmless. Not only does this improve your overall health and well-being, but it also improves your exercise capacity. There is a reduction in postexercise muscle inflammation (with an associated decrease in delayed onset muscle soreness), helping to repair bodily tissues and speed recovery.

While there are dozens of known antioxidants, four of them are absolutely indispensable: vitamin C, vitamin E, coenzyme Q10, and alpha-lipoic acid. These antioxidants work synergistically with one another; their combined effect is greater than the sum of their individual actions. Other antioxidants that are beneficial include selenium, lycopene, isoflavones, and polyphenols (although they don't have the synergistic capabilities of the "big four").

It is virtually impossible, however, to consume adequate quantities of antioxidants from food sources. For example, you'd have to drink eleven glasses of orange juice in order to get the recommended amount of vitamin C. Hence, supplementation is an absolute necessity. Table 10.1 lists the major antioxidants with corresponding dosages.

As a rule, it is best to consume supplements in conjunction with a meal. The absorption of micronutrients is improved when they are consumed with food. This also improves gastrointestinal tolerance of the supplement.

TABLE 10.1

Antioxidant	Dosage
Vitamin C	800 mg
Vitamin E	600 IU
Coenzyme Q10	50 mg
Alpha-lipoic acid	100 mg
Polyphenols	50 mg
Soy isoflavones	50 mg
Lycopene	10 mg
Selenium	200 mcg

IU = International Units.

Cheat a Little

Throughout the ages, food always has been a source of great temptation. Dating all the way back to Adam and Eve, there was the forbidden fruit; that luscious apple was simply too much to resist. Today, with food so plentiful, the temptations are literally endless. Let's face it, a great deal of willpower is required to pass up a slice of birthday cake or forgo a bucket of chicken wings. For some, the thought of never again eating these types of foods is too much to bear. After several months of deprivation, they break down and go on an eating binge, scarfing down everything in sight.

To help keep your sanity, it is acceptable—even beneficial—to have a "cheat" day. On your cheat day, you can eat basically anything you want, including sugar and/or fat-laden foods. Within reason, there are no restrictions. Go ahead and order a pizza. Frequent your favorite fast-food restaurant. Have a candy bar. Whatever you heart desires, feel free to indulge. You don't need to feel guilty about cheating; consider it a reward for sticking to your diet.

Try not to go too far overboard, though. While a little overindulgence won't have any effect on your physique, consuming mass quantities of food very well could (and it also can make you pretty sick!). Accordingly, don't allow the total calories on your cheat day to exceed more than 150 percent of your estimated daily intake. For instance, if you normally eat 1600 calories, don't go past 2400 calories. This will give you plenty of leeway to satisfy your food cravings while keeping caloric intake within a reasonable range.

Finally, make sure to limit cheating to no more than one day per week. Try to pick a specific cheat day and stay with it. Regimentation is an important part of maintaining a healthy lifestyle, and when cheating becomes a habit, regimentation goes by the wayside. Stick with the program and make your cheat day a special treat.

RECIPES OF THE TOP FITNESS MODELS

You really can eat healthy foods that actually taste great! Just because a dish is low in fat and sugar doesn't mean that it has to be bland.

I asked some of the top fitness models in the world—women who make their living by looking great—to submit their favorite healthy recipes. On the following pages are their mouth-watering responses. You'll find everything from breakfast, lunch, and dinner entrées to protein shakes and snacks. And, best of all, most of the recipes take only minutes to prepare!

So go ahead and indulge yourself. Eat like a champion and enjoy!

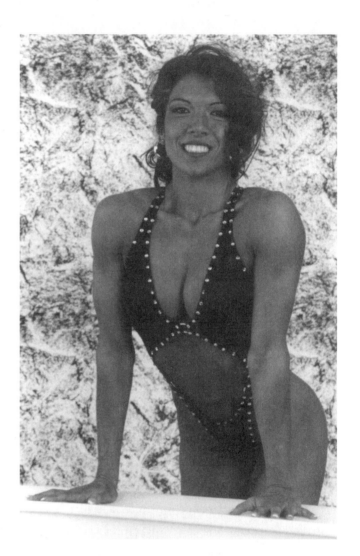

SUSIE CURRY
Fitness International Champion
c/o JMP Management
P.O. Box 293
Presto, PA 15412

⬅ SUSIE'S CHICKEN AND BEAN SALAD SUPREME ⬅

Ingredients:

1 medium bowl of romaine and iceberg lettuce
¼ cup of red kidney beans
¼ cup of garbanzo beans
½ cup of steamed chicken (cut into small pieces)
1 tablespoon of almond slivers
3 tablespoons of olive oil and vinegar

Directions:

Chop up lettuce into pieces and place in large bowl. Add beans and chicken and toss together until thoroughly mixed. Top with almonds and oil/vinegar combination and enjoy!

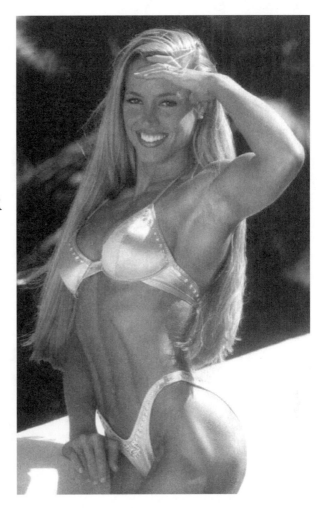

SHONNA MCCARVER
Ms. Galaxy,
Physique Champion
P.O. Box 19501
Houston, TX 77224
http://www.shonna.com

☞ SHONNA'S STRAWBERRY DELIGHT ☜

Ingredients:

1 ¼ cups water
⅛ cup strawberry nectar
3 frozen strawberries
2 tablespoons sugar-free vanilla pudding
1 ½ scoops whey protein
4 cubes of ice

Directions:

Put water, strawberry nectar, and strawberries in a blender and puree for about ten seconds. Add in protein, pudding, and ice and blend on high until mixture has a smooth consistency. Pour into tall glass and enjoy!

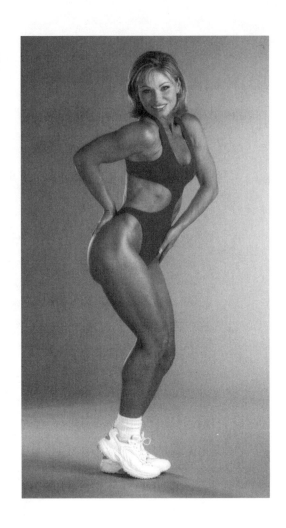

TAMILEE WEBB
Ms. "Buns of Steel"
P.O. Box 676107
Rancho Santa Fe, CA 92067
www.Tamileewebb.com

☞ TAMILEE'S PROVINCIAL TURKEY ☜

Ingredients:

4 ounces turkey breast (cubed)
1 cup kidney beans
1 cup chickpea salad
1 cup peppers,
1 cup celery
1 cup tomatoes
1 cup scallions

Directions:

Combine all ingredients in large salad bowl. Add herbs to taste, toss, and enjoy!

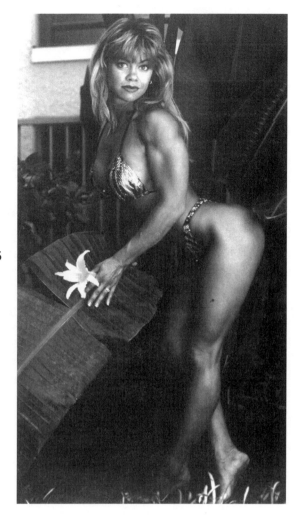

MARLA DUNCAN
Ms. Fitness USA
1911 Douglas Blvd. Suite 85 PMB 345
Roseville, CA 95661
www.marladuncan.com

☞ MARLA'S MULTIBEAN STEW ☜

Ingredients:

2 15-ounce cans red kidney beans
1 15-ounce can garbanzo beans
2 ½ cups water
2 medium potatoes, peeled,
   quartered lengthwise, and sliced
1 cup thinly sliced carrot
½ cup chopped onion

6-ounce can tomato paste
2 teaspoons chili powder
1 teaspoon salt
1 teaspoon dried basil, crushed
¼ teaspoon garlic powder
¼ teaspoon pepper
8 ounces lowfat jack cheese

Directions:

In a Dutch oven combine undrained kidney beans and garbanzo beans, water, potatoes, carrot, onion, tomato paste, chili powder, salt, basil, and pepper and bring to boil. Reduce heat, cover, and simmer 30 minutes until veggies are tender. Top with cheese and enjoy!

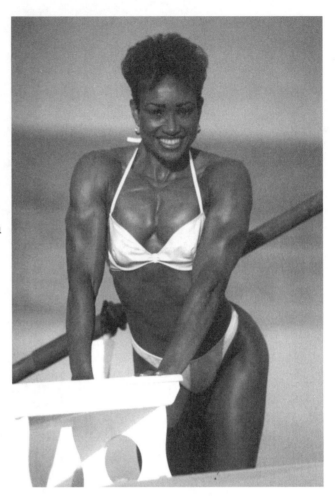

LISA LOWE
NPC Fitness Universe Champion
1250-I Newell Avenue, #234
Walnut Creek, CA 94596
www.lisalowefitness.com

⮞ LISA'S CAJUN CHILI ⮜

Ingredients:

1 pound lean ground skinless turkey
1 large onion, chopped
16-ounce can stewed tomatoes (no salt)
16-ounce can tomato sauce (no salt)
3 garlic cloves, crushed
2 tablespoons chili powder
1½ teaspoon cumin
1½ teaspoon dried oregano leaves
½ teaspoon red pepper flakes
pinch garlic powder

Directions:

Cook the ground turkey, garlic powder, onion, and bell peppers over medium heat. Add cumin and chili powder, mixing well. Add stewed tomatoes, tomato sauce, oregano, pepper flakes, and crushed garlic. Heat to a boil. Cover and simmer for thirty minutes. Serve over brown rice or enjoy by itself!

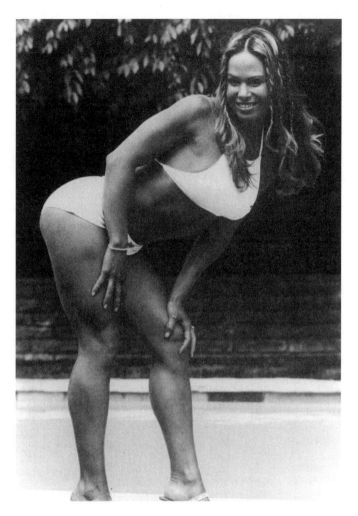

AMY FADHLI
Fitness America Champion
P.O. Box 25095
Los Angeles, CA 90025
www.afadhli.com

⌒ AMY'S BREAKFAST SCRAMBLE ⌒

Ingredients:

   6 egg whites and 1 yolk
   3 mushrooms, diced
   ½ small tomato, diced
   ½ cup shredded fat-free cheese
   2 thin slices of turkey breast, diced

Directions:

   Preheat a nonstick skillet at 350 degrees. Scramble egg whites, mushrooms, tomato, and turkey together in a large bowl and pour into heated skillet. Cook to taste. Top with fat-free cheese and enjoy!

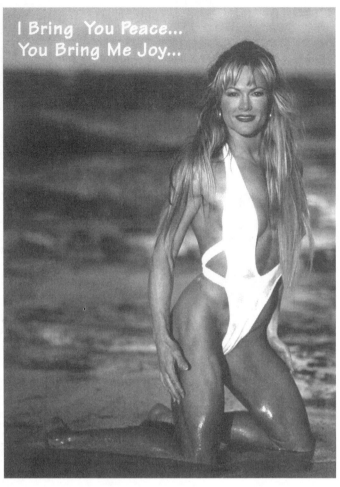

LORI ANN LLOYD
Extreme Fitness
Champion
LoriStar Productions
P.O. Box 561355
Orlando, FL 32856-1355
www.loriannlloyd.com

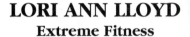

LORI ANN'S TURKEY BREAST TORTILLAS

Ingredients:

1 pound ground turkey breast
½ cup oatmeal
½ cup barbeque sauce (your favorite type)
1 whole egg
1 whole wheat tortilla
1 teaspoon soy cheddar cheese
½ tomato diced
salt and pepper to taste

Directions:

Mix ingredients in bowl. Heat skillet to medium low. Shape patties in your hand and carefully place in pan. Use cooking spray to avoid sticking. Cook covered for about 5 minutes; then turn them over, cooking until done. Place in tortilla, topping with cheese and tomato, and enjoy!

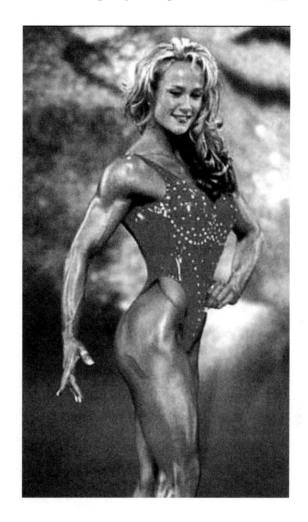

LENA JOHANNESEN
European Fitness Champion
P.O. Box 325
Culver City, CA 90232
www.lenajohannesen.com

☞　**LENA'S HEALTHY BURGERS**　☜

Ingredients:

2 garlic cloves, minced
3 tablespoons fresh mint, chopped
1½ cups non/lowfat yogurt
1½ pounds ground turkey, lean
2 teaspoons feta cheese, crumbled
6 pita bread loaves, sliced
1½ red onions, sliced

Directions:

Combine garlic and mint in a small bowl and mash. Add yogurt, mix and set aside. Combine turkey and feta cheese in mixing bowl. Form into 8 patties and sprinkle with pepper. Broil 5–10 minutes, per side or until turkey is cooked through. Serve in pita bread with tomatoes, onions, and yogurt sauce, and enjoy!

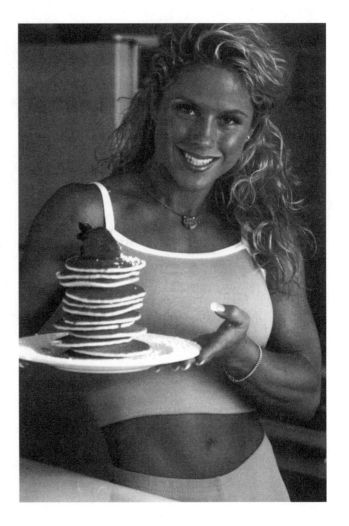

MONICA BRANT
Fitness Olympia Champion
333 Washington Blvd.
Manna Del Rey, CA 90292
www.monicabrant.com

≈ **MONICA'S POWER PANCAKES** ≈

Ingredients:

4–5 egg whites
3 ounces low-fat tofu
¼ cup nonfat cottage cheese
⅓ cup Coach's oats
dash of unsweetened soy milk
pinch of cinnamon
¼ teaspoon vanilla and/or almond extract
For a berry flavor, add ½ scoop of strawberry or other fruit-flavored
protein powder

Directions:

Preheat nonstick griddle to 400 degrees. Place all ingredients in a blender and blend until a smooth consistency is achieved. Spray griddle with cooking spray and pour batter onto griddle in 4-inch pools. Brown lightly on both sides. Top with low-fat butter and/or sugar-free syrup and enjoy!

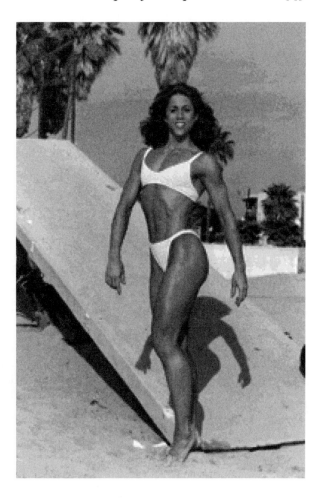

AMANDA DOERRER
IFBB Fitness Pro
P.O. Box 230487
Encinitas, CA 92023-0487
www.amandadoerrer.co

☞ AMANDA'S FAT-FREE FETA PIZZA ☜

Ingredients:

whole wheat fat-free pitas
fat-free feta cheese
fat-free mozarella cheese
fat-free parmesan cheese
1 cup diced tomatoes
½ chopped green onions
dash of minced garlic, basil, oregano, rosemary

Directions:

Spray cookie sheet or pizza pan with nonstick cooking spray. Cut fat-free pitas into triangle wedges and arrange on pan. Spread diced tomatoes and onions on each piece. Sprinkle with cheeses and spices to taste. Bake in oven at 325 for about 10 minutes or until cheese is melted. (*Hint:* Use a lower shelf in your oven so the cheese does not turn into a big glob.) Serve either as a hot appetizer or as a meal and enjoy!

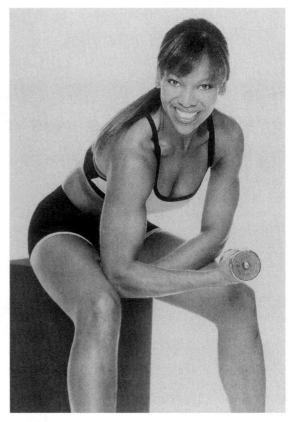

DONNA RICHARDSON
National Aerobics Champion
www.donnarichardson.com

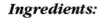 **DONNA'S SEAFOOD NORFOLK**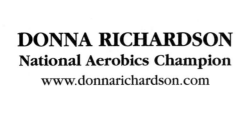

Ingredients:

2 carrots, sliced
1 onion, chopped
¼ cup flour
½ teaspoon salt, divided
¼ teaspoon pepper, divided
½ lb. shrimp
½ lb. sea scallops

1 teaspoon lemon zest
2 tablespoons lemon juice
Butter replacement, such as Butter
   Buds, equal to 1/4 pound butter
⅔ cup white wine
2 tablespoons capers
6 oz. lump crab meat

Directions:

Coat large skillet with nonstick cooking spray. Over medium heat, add carrots and onion; cook until tender, 8-10 minutes; adding ½ tablespoon water, if necessary, to prevent sticking. Remove vegetables to plate and set aside. In small bowl, combine flour, ¼ tsp. salt, ⅛ tsp. pepper. Toss shrimp and scallops in flour mixture. Recoat skillet with cooking spray. Over medium heat cook shrimp and scallops until almost cooked through and lightly browned; remove to plate. In small bowl combine zest, juice, butter replacement, wine and capers. Add to skillet and cook, scraping up brown bits from the bottom of skillet until thickened, about 2-3 minutes. Add crab meat, reserved vegetables, shrimp and scallops and remaining salt and pepper. Bring to a boil and cook 1 minute. Enjoy!

MORE HEALTHY RECIPES

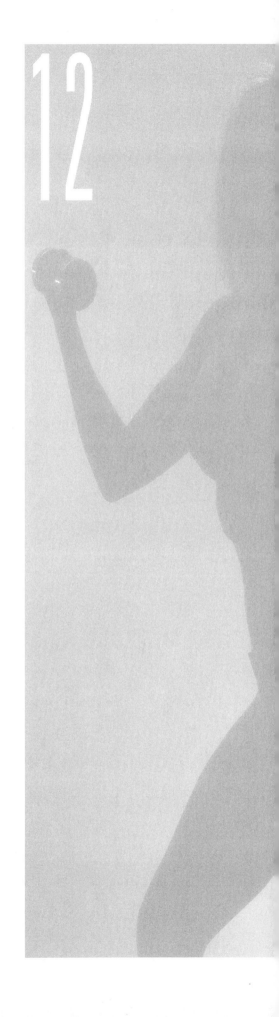

On the following pages are some of my own favorite healthy recipes. For convenience, I have categorized them into breakfast, lunch, dinner, and snacks. Feel free to experiment and add your own twists to these recipes. If you get creative, there's no limit to what you can come up with!

Breakfast

⌒ BANANA/OATMEAL DELIGHT ⌒

Ingredients:

2 ripe bananas—mashed

1 cup oatmeal

¼ cup whole wheat flour or cream of wheat

1 cup of water combined by a whisk with ¼ cup powdered egg whites

2 teaspoons of brown sugar

1 teaspoon nutmeg

1 teaspoon cinnamon

1 teaspoon ground cloves

1 teaspoon ginger

Directions:

In mixing bowl, combine all ingredients and mix them together. Spray a loaf pan with non-stick cooking spray and pour in ingredients. Insert a toothpick into center of mix. Bake at 350 degrees for 45 minutes or until toothpick comes out clean and enjoy!

⌒ WHOLE WHEAT CINNAMON RAISIN BREAD ⌒

Ingredients:

8 egg whites

4 cups water

1 teaspoon nutmeg

1 teaspoon cinnamon

¼ cup honey

1 lb raisins

2 cups powdered lecithin

2 teaspoons baking powder

2 ½ lbs whole wheat flour

Directions:

In large mixing bowl, combine eggs, spices, and honey with 1 cup water and mix until blended. Add 2 more cups water, raisins, lecithin, and baking powder and continue mixing. Add final cup water and sift in flour while mixing thoroughly.

Separate dough into 4 equal components and place in non-stick baking pan. Bake at 300 degrees for 1 hour or until top is golden brown and enjoy!

↪ MEXICAN EGG-WHITE OMELETTE ↩

Ingredients:

6 egg whites
2 tablespoons medium salsa
1 slice fat-free cheese

Directions:

Spray frying pan with non-stick cooking spray. Add egg whites and pull at edges until solid. Place cheese and salsa on top, fold over, and enjoy!

↪ POWER PANCAKES ↩

Ingredients:

1 cup Aunt Jemima Complete whole wheat pancake mix
1 cup water
1 scoop whey protein

Directions:

Preheat a griddle at 400 degrees and spray with non-stick cooking spray. Combine ingredients into a mixing bowl. Pour ingredients onto griddle in 8 equal circles. Flip after approximately 30 seconds. Serve with all-fruit jelly and enjoy!

↪ CINNAMON NUT MUSELI ↩

Ingredients:

3 cups rolled oats
$\frac{1}{4}$ cup chopped walnuts
1 teaspoon cinnamon
$\frac{1}{8}$ cup raisins
$\frac{1}{4}$ cup chopped hazelnuts
$\frac{1}{4}$ cup wheatgerm
$\frac{1}{4}$ cup skim milk

Directions:

Combine ingredients into a large bowl, mix together, and enjoy.

☞ APRICOT/WALNUT OATMEAL ☜

Ingredients:

1 cup oatmeal
¾ cup water
6 dried apricots
⅛ cup chopped walnuts
1 tablespoon nutmeg

Directions:

Place oatmeal in bowl and add water. Microwave oatmeal according to directions on package. Add apricots, walnuts, and nutmeg and enjoy!

☞ EGG WHITE MCBAGEL ☜

Ingredients:

1 whole wheat bagel
4 egg whites
2 slices fat-free cheese (any kind)
1 teaspoon basil
1 teaspoon oregano
2 tablespoons canned roasted bell peppers

Directions:

Cut bagel in half and toast until golden brown. Spray non-stick frying pan with PAM and heat at 350 degrees. Pour egg whites into pan and cook omelet style, adding oregano, basil, and bell peppers during cooking. When eggs are no longer "watery," top with cheese and fold. Place egg on bagel and enjoy!

~ *Lunch* ~

⤳ MULTI-FRUIT SEAFOOD SALAD ⤳

Ingredients:

$\frac{1}{2}$ large pineapple

3 mandarin oranges

3 kiwis

$\frac{1}{2}$ head Romaine lettuce

1 $\frac{1}{2}$ cups cooked shrimp, crab, or tuna

Directions:

Cut pineapple, oranges, and kiwis into small cubes and place in large bowl. Add seafood into bowl. Toss with salad greens and enjoy!

⤳ MEGA-VITAMIN VEGETABLE SOUP ⤳

Ingredients:

32-ounce can tomato soup

64 ounces water

12-ounce can tomato paste

10 bouillon cubes

2 tablespoons garlic

3 tablespoons Italian seasoning

16 ounces squash

16 ounces broccoli

16 ounces green beans

16 ounces cauliflower

16 ounces carrots

Directions:

Combine tomato soup, tomato paste, water and, bouillon in large pot and stir over a medium heat until blended. Add garlic and seasoning as you stir.

Chop vegetables into small cubes and add to the mix. Heat for approximately 15 minutes, or until vegetables are soft, and enjoy!

☞ Fat-Free Tuna Melt ☜

Ingredients:

1 can albacore tuna
2 slices Healthy Choice fat-free cheese
2 slices whole wheat bread

Directions:

Open tuna and put half of contents on each slice of bread. Place cheese on top of each slice. Bake at 450 degrees until cheese melts and enjoy!

☞ Chicken Caeser Salad ☜

Ingredients:

6 ounces chicken breast
1/2 head romaine lettuce
1 tablespoon fat-free Caeser dressing
1 tablespoon Ms. Dash

Directions:

Cut chicken into small strips. Place chicken in large bowl with lettuce and toss well. Sprinkle on Ms. Dash and dressing. Toss again and enjoy!

☞ Zucchini-Squash Salad ☜

Ingredients:

1 medium zucchini
1 medium yellow squash
2 teaspoons Dijon mustard
1 teaspoon balsamic vinegar
1/2 teaspoon crushed black pepper
1 teaspoon light soy sauce

Directions:

Cut zucchini and squash into juliene strips and place in a large bowl. Combine remaining ingredients in a mixing bowl and blend together until smooth. Pour mixture over squash and zucchini. Toss until evenly mixed throughout and enjoy!

☞ POTATO/VINAGRETTE CHICKEN SALAD ☜

Ingredients:

1 large yam
4 ounces green beans
1 tablespoon extra virgin olive oil
6 ounces chicken breast cut into cubes
¼ cup no-fat vinagrette dressing
6 ounces chopped romaine lettuce

Directions:

In large pot, boil 16 ounces of water. Cut yams into quarters and place them in boiling water. After 3 minutes, add green beans and boil for another 4 minutes.

Preheat a separate pan and spray with Pam, then add chicken and cook for about 6 minutes or until the meat is no longer pink. Place all ingredients in large salad bowl, add vinagrette dressing, and enjoy!

Dinner

LEMON/CAYENNE RED SNAPPER

Ingredients:

1 pound red snapper
½ lemon
¼ teaspoon garlic powder
¼ teaspoon onion powder
¼ teaspoon paprica
¼ teaspoon cayenne pepper

Directions:

Place fish on broiler pan. Squeeze juice of lemon over fish. Add garlic, onion, paprika, and pepper. Broil for approximately 10 minutes. Serve over a bed of steamed rice and enjoy!

GROUND TURKEY SUPREME

Ingredients:

1 pound 99% fat-free ground turkey or chicken
10 ounces frozen chopped spinach, thawed
1 tablespoon low-sodium ketchup
1 tablespoon basil
1 tablespoon garlic powder
¼ cup chopped onion
¼ cup chopped red pepper
2 tablespoons Dijon mustard
1 teaspoon honey

Directions:

In mixing bowl, combine all ingredients except mustard and honey. Spray a loaf pan with PAM cooking spray and pour in ingredients. Bake at 350 degrees for 45 minutes or until toothpick comes out clean. Glaze over with mustard and honey. Bake another 10 minutes and enjoy!

☞ LOW-FAT FIBER-RICH FRIED RICE ☜

Ingredients:

2 cups cooked brown rice
3 egg whites
½ cup peas
4 ounces cooked chicken breasts cut into small pieces
½ cup bean sprouts
½ cup bamboo shoots
1 tablespoon low-sodium soy sauce

Directions:

Spray a saute pan with non-stick cooking spray and scramble egg whites until firm. Set aside for future use. Re-spray pan with non-stick cooking spray and saute bean sprouts, bamboo shoots, and peas until heated. Set aside for future use. Re-spray pan with non-stick cooking spray and add rice, cooking until rice starts to brown. Add in egg whites, chicken breast, bean sprouts, bamboo shoots, and soy sauce. Mix well and enjoy!

☞ TEX-MEX TURKEY CHEESEBURGER ☜

Ingredients:

6 ounces ground turkey breast
2 tablespoons medium salsa
1 slice fat-free cheese
1 whole wheat bun

Directions:

Pat down turkey into a pate and place on grill. After flipping, place cheese on top. When cheese melts, place on bun and garnish with salsa. Enjoy!

LOW FAT CHICKEN BURRITO

Ingredients:

8 ounces grilled, skinless chicken breast
1 ounce shredded fat-free cheddar cheese
1 low-fat flour burrito
¼ cup fat-free salsa

Directions:

Preheat a frying pan and spray with non-stick cooking spray. Place tortilla in the pan until warm. Place the cheese evenly on top of the tortilla and then combine chicken and salsa over the cheese. Fold each 1-inch border over the center and pin them together with your fingers. Flip the bottom lip of the tortilla up and over, and then push the lip over the burrito so that all the ingredients are contained. Heat for 3 minutes on each side and enjoy!

LEMON PEPPER SWORDFISH

Ingredients:

8 ounces swordfish steak
3 tablespoons lemon juice
1 teaspoon oregano
1 teaspoon pepper
1 teaspoon lemon/herb spice

Directions:

Place swordfish in a large bowl and combine lemon juice, oregano, pepper, and lemon/herb spice on top. Mix ingredients and let marinate for 1 hour. Place swordfish on barbecue. Let stand for 5 minutes and turn over for another 5 minutes. Serve with salad or brown rice and enjoy!

⤠ PEPPERED STEAK ⤟

Ingredients:

8 ounces sirloin steak
⅛ cup light soy sauce
3 teaspoons ground black pepper
⅛ cup balsamic vinegar

Directions:

Trim all visible fat from steak. Combine steak with remaining ingredients and place in a self-closing plastic bag. Refrigerate for 1 hour. Remove steak from marinade and grill at a high flame. Cook to taste and enjoy!

⤠ CHICKEN CACCIATORE ⤟

Ingredients:

2 skinless chicken breasts
½ onion sliced into rings
1 teaspoon garlic
½ can (14 oz) chopped tomatoes
8 ounces low-sodium marinara sauce
½ teaspoon of oregano
½ teaspoon of basil
8 ounces angel hair pasta, boiled al dente

Directions:

Spray cooking pan with non-stick cooking spray. Put chicken into pan and brown over at medium height. Remove chicken and set aside. Re-coat pan with non-stick cooking spray and add all ingredients except chicken and pasta. Cook at medium heat for 7 minutes. Add chicken to the mix and simmer on low heat for 20 minutes. Pour chicken and sauce over pasta and enjoy!

☞ GARLIC SHRIMP-KA-BOB ☜

Ingredients:

8 ounces large shrimp
8 cherry tomatoes
½ green pepper cut into strips
1 tablespoon garlic
1 teaspoon ground pepper
½ teaspoon of oregano
½ teaspoon of basil
2 tablespoons balsamic vinegar

Directions:

Combine garlic, ground pepper, oregano, basil, and balsamic vinegar into a large bowl. Marinate shrimp, tomatoes, and green pepper in the mix for 1 hour. Place shrimp, tomatoes, and green pepper on skewers and barbeque until slightly brown. Remove from the skewers and enjoy!

☞ TURKEY TETRAZZINI ☜

Ingredients:

4 ounces angel hair pasta cooked al dente
8 ounces skinless chicken breast cut into cubes
1 tablespoon onion powder
1 tablespoon light soy sauce
¼ teaspoon ground pepper
½ teaspoon of oregano
½ teaspoon of paprika
¼ pound chopped mushrooms

Directions:

Spray a large cooking pan with non-stick cooking spray. Combine chicken, onions, and oregano into pan and cook on medium heat for about 15 minutes.

Remove chicken , add remaining ingredients to pan with ½ cup of water, and cook for 5 minutes over medium heat. Pour back in chicken mixture and saute until slightly brown. Place chicken mixture over pasta and enjoy!

⌒ SEA BASS MARSALA ⌒

Ingredients:

8 ounces sea bass fillets
1 tablespoon onion powder
½ cup marsala wine
1 tablespoon oregano

Directions:

Combine wine, onion powder, and oregano with enough water to fill 2 inches of a large saucepan and bring liquid to a boil. Arrange fish on a steaming tray and place on a rack about an inch above the liquid. Cover and steam for about 15 minutes and enjoy!

⌒ CHICKEN DIVAN ⌒

Ingredients:

1 pound of fresh broccoli
12 ounces skinless chicken, sliced into strips
4 tablespoons fat-free Parmesan cheese
10 ounces low-sodium chicken soup
⅓ cup water

Directions:

Preheat oven to 375 degrees. Arrange broccoli in layers over chicken in baking dish. Sprinkle Parmesan cheese over broccoli and chicken. Mix soup with water and heat and pour over contents. Bake 20 to 30 minutes and enjoy!

MEDITERRANEAN BROILED SOLE

Ingredients:

8 ounces sole fillets
1 egg white
2 tablespoons lemon juice
1 chopped garlic clove
¼ cup whole wheat bread crumbs
¼ cup no-fat grated Parmesan cheese

Directions:

Spray non-stick frying pan with PAM and heat at 400 degrees. Pour egg whites and lemon into a bowl and mix thoroughly. Place remaining ingredients except fish in another bowl and mix. Dip fish fillets in egg whites and then dip in bread crumb mixture. Place fillets in broiling pan and broil until lightly brown on each side. When finished, serve with salad and enjoy!

Snacks

☞ PROTEIN-POWERED ORANGE WHIP ☜

Ingredients:

- 1 ½ packets unflavored gelatin
- 3 ½ cups orange juice
- 3 tablespoons lemon juice
- 2 tablespoons frozen apple juice
- 2 packets artificial sweetener
- 1 scoop whey protein powder

Directions:

In mixing bowl, combine ½ cup orange juice with gelatin. In separate pot, heat remaining orange juice, bringing it to a boil. Add orange juice to gelatin mixture and stir until gelatin is dissolved. Add apple juice, lemon juice, artificial sweetener, and whey protein powder. Chill in refrigerator until mixture thickens. Beat with mixer until fluffy and enjoy!

☞ ORANGE CREAMSICLE PROTEIN DRINK ☜

Ingredients:

- 1 scoop french vanilla whey protein
- 1 packet orange Crystal Lite
- 12 ounces water

Directions:

Combine ingredients in a tall glass. Stir and enjoy!

☞ RASPBERRY MET-RX PUDDING ☜

Ingredients:

- 1 packet vanilla Met-Rx
- 4 ounces raspberry seltzer

Directions:

Pour seltzer into a cup and add Met-Rx. Stir until smooth and creamy and enjoy!

☞ PROTEIN-POWERED VANILLA COFFEE ☜

Ingredients:

8 ounces of brewed coffee

1 scoop whey protein

1 tablespoon fat-free milk (if desired)

1 packet sugar substitute (if desired)

Directions:

Pour coffee into an oversized coffee cup. Add ingredients and enjoy!

☞ BLACK BEAN SALSA ☜

Ingredients:

2 cups black beans

1 teaspoon onion powder

1 medium tomato (diced)

1 small jalepeno pepper (diced)

$\frac{1}{2}$ cup lemon juice

3 tablespoons balsamic vinegar

1 teaspoon Ms. Dash

Directions:

Place all ingredients except for the black beans in a food processor and blend until thick (don't liquefy). Pour mixture over beans in a large bowl and stir well. Chill overnight in refrigerator and enjoy!

☞ VANILLA PROTEIN SMOOTHIE ☜

Ingredients:

1 cup skim milk

1 scoop French vanilla whey protein powder

1 teaspoon vanilla extract

3 or 4 ice cubes

Directions:

Combine ingredients into blender and blend at high speed until a smooth consistency is achieved. Pour into tall glass and enjoy!

⤙ CURRY DIP ⤚

Ingredients:

1 medium tomato sliced into quarters

1 tablespoon curry powder

1 onion (sliced)

8 ounces non-fat cottage cheese

¼ teaspoon Ms. Dash

Directions:

Place ingredients in blender and process on high speed until thoroughly blended. Serve with raw vegetables and enjoy!

⤙ VANILLA CREME FRAPPUCHINO ⤚

Ingredients:

2 cups water

2 teaspoons instant coffee

1 scoop French vanilla whey protein powder

1 teaspoon vanilla extract

1 teaspoon cinnamon

3 or 4 ice cubes

Directions:

Place all ingredients except ice cubes and cinnamon in a blender and puree until thoroughly mixed. Add ice cubes and blend on high until a smooth consistency is achieved. Top with cinnamon and enjoy!

Appendix A
HIGH FIBER FOODS

FOOD	AMOUNT	FIBER CONTENT (G)
Apple	Medium	3
All bran cereal	1 ounce	10
Barley	1 cup	6
Blackberries	1 cup	8
Black beans	1 cup	19
Bread (whole wheat)	2 slices	6
Broccoli	1 cup	8
Chick peas	1 cup	12
Corn	Medium	5
Green peas	1 cup	18
Lentils	1 cup	15
Oatmeal	1 cup	4
Pear	Medium	4
Raspberries	1 cup	9
Rice (brown)	1 cup	5
Spinach	1 cup	7
Yams	Medium	7

Appendix B
GLOSSARY OF TERMS

Adipocyte. Fat cell.

Aerobic Exercise. Any activity that allows your body to consistently replenish oxygen to your working muscles. It is performed at a low to moderate intensity and is endurance-oriented. Both fat and glycogen are burned for fuel.

Alpha-2 Receptor. The "entrance" that allows fat to enter an adipocyte.

Anaerobic Exercise. Any activity that utilizes oxygen at a faster rate than your body can replenish it in the working muscles. This type of exercise is intense and short in duration. Glycogen is the primary source of fuel.

Barbell. A long bar, usually about 6 feet in length, that can accommodate weighted plates on each end. The Olympic barbell is the industry standard and weighs 45 pounds.

Bench. An apparatus designed for performing exercises in a seated or lying position. Many benches are adjustable so that exercises can be performed at a wide array of different angles.

Beta Receptor. The "exit" that allows fat to escape from an adipocyte.

Bodysculpting. The art of shaping your muscles to optimal proportions.

Cardio. Short for cardiovascular (aerobic) exercise.

Circuit Training. A series of exercise machines set up in sequence. The exercises are performed one after the other, each stressing a different muscle group.

Collar. A clamp that secures weighted plates on a barbell or dumbbell.

Compound Movement. An exercise that involves two or more joints in the performance of the movement. Examples include squats, bench presses, and chins.

Contraction. Shortening a muscle.

Cross Training. Using two or more different exercises in a routine, generally in the context of aerobic activities.

Definition. The absence of fat in the presence of well-developed muscle.

Dumbbell. A shortened version of a barbell, usually about 12 inches long, that allows an exercise to be performed one arm at a time.

Estrogen. A primary female hormone, linked to increased fat storage.

Exercise. An individual movement intended to tax muscular function.

Failure. The point in an exercise where you cannot physically perform another rep.

Flexibility. A litheness of the joints, muscle, and connective tissue that dictates range of motion.

Form. The technique utilized in performing the biomechanics of an exercise.

Free Weights. Barbells and dumbbells, as opposed to exercise machines.

Giant Set. A series of three or more exercises performed in succession without any rest between sets.

Hypertrophy. An increase in muscle mass.

Intensity. The amount of effort involved in a set.

Isolation Movement. An exercise that involves only one joint in the performance of the movement. Examples include cable crossovers, biceps curls, and leg extensions.

Nautilus. A brand of exercise equipment found in many health clubs. The term has become synonymous with any exercise machine.

Plates. Flat, round weights that can be place at the end of a barbell or dumbbell.

Progesterone. A primary female hormone, linked to increased appetite.

Pump. The pooling of blood in a muscle due to intense anaerobic exercise.

Repetition (Rep). One complete movement of an exercise.

Resistance. The amount of weight used in an exercise.

Rest Interval. The amount of rest time taken between sets.

Routine. The configuration of exercises, sets, and reps that one utilizes in a training session.

Set. A series of repetitions performed in succession.

Symmetry. The way in which muscle groups complement one another, creating a proportional physique.

Testosterone. A hormone that is responsible for promoting muscle mass.

Thermogenesis. Increased body heat, which accelerates fat burning.